D0044823

The Carnitine Miracle

The Carnitine Miracle

The Supernutrient Program That Promotes High Energy, Fat Burning, Heart Health, Brain Wellness, and Longevity

Robert Crayhon, M.S.

M. Evans and Company, Inc.
New York

Copyright © 1998 Robert Crayhon
All rights reserved. No part of this book may be reproduced or transmitted in any form or by any means without the written permission of the publisher.

M. Evans and Company, Inc.
216 East 49th Street
New York, NY 10017

Library of Congress Cataloging-in-Publication Data

Crayhon, Robert, 1961–
    The carnitine miracle : the supernutrient that promotes high energy, weight loss, heart health, brain wellness, and longevity / Robert Crayhon.
        p. cm.
    Includes bibliographical references and index.
    ISBN 0-87131-825-3 (cloth)
    1. Carnitine—Health aspects. 2. Carnitine—Therapeutic use. 3. Carnitine deficiency. I. Title.
QP772.C3C73   1998
613.2'8—dc21   98-9723

DESIGNED AND TYPESET BY RIK LAIN SCHELL

Manufactured in the United States of America

9 8 7 6 5

ATTENTION

The advice offered in this book, although based on the author's experience with many thousands of patients, is not intended to be a substitute for the advice and counsel of your personal physician.

For Kristin

ACKNOWLEDGMENTS

I would like to thank the many nutrition experts who have shared their thoughts with me during the writing of this book: Leigh Broadhurst, Lee Carter, Clara Felix, Parris Kidd, Richard Kunin, Brian Leibovitz, Barbara Marquette, Mark McCarty, Jeffrey Moss, Dileep Sachan and Jerry Schlesser. Linda Lizotte did a great job offering helpful comments during the preparation of the final manuscript. I am particularly indebted to Loren Cordain for sharing his thoughts with me as I went through his Paleolithic nutrition library and for helping me sharpen the Paleolithic section of this book.

I would also like to thank Sue Radcliffe for her sharp eye and invaluable help during the final preparation of this manuscript. Her proofreading gifts and her many valuable comments allowed me to bring my thoughts to you with the utmost clarity.

I would also like to thank my clients, who through the years have taught me more about carnitine and the power of Paleolithic nutrition than anyone else.

CONTENTS

FOREWORD

As a researcher, clinician, and educator in the field of nutrition for the past twenty years, I continue to be astounded by the rapid growth of knowledge in this field—knowledge from both the scientific journals and the clinical breakthroughs of practitioners. What excites me is that both of these areas are important. What disappoints me is that so few nutritionists seem to be familiar with both.

Robert Crayhon is an exception. He is an outstanding scholar as well as an experienced clinician, and he brings both of these important strengths to bear in creating one of the most important nutrition books of recent times—*The Carnitine Miracle*. This remarkable book covers a lot of territory, and does so with clarity, brevity, and always with a sense of the clinical bottom line.

But why carnitine?

Carnitine is a remarkable nutrient that the body needs to make energy, and energy is the most important health-promoting force in the body. Carnitine is also a crucial heart-supporting nutrient. It is probably the most important nutrient to use for promoting weight loss. A special form of carnitine known as acetyl-L-carnitine has been found to slow the progression of Alzheimer's disease and promote overall brain wellness. And, as Robert shows, carnitine has also been found helpful in treating a wide range of other health problems.

I am glad there is finally a book on this remarkable nutrient, and one that comes from someone who has spent the last twelve years both researching carnitine and using it in his clinical practice. Robert Crayhon has more experience with carnitine than anyone I know, and there is no one better to break the carnitine story. Armed with Robert's book, you can now unlock the power of this nutrient to help you lose weight, promote heart health, maximize brain health, and enhance your energy and overall well-being.

Yet this is more than just a book about the nutrient carnitine. It features a brilliant and succinct discussion of the Paleolithic diet—what humans ate for 2.6 million years. There are many important nutritional lessons to be learned from studying this wide expanse of human nutrition, most notably: don't be afraid of protein, and do be afraid of modern refined foods. *The Carnitine Miracle* also discusses the benefits of eating both the right kinds and amounts of carbohydrates, fats, and protein. Robert's discussion of these dietary elements is excellent, and forms the background upon which he creates his eating plan, the Carnitine Program.

I am excited that Americans are interested in taking supplements and improving the quality of their diet. These are important strategies for disease prevention and enhancing quality of life. Yet how practical are the suggestions? How well will the patient follow the advice? And, most important of all, how well does the patient feel thirty to sixty days after starting the program?

While some in the health field claim to have achieved impressive results with strict nutritional regimes, few patients are able to follow them. What I appreciate about Robert's work as a clinician and author is that his suggestions are reasonable, easy to follow, and based on his work with actual patients. His assertion that carnitine and a diet based on Paleolithic Principles enhances health is not merely a theory; it is backed by his own vast clinical experience as well as the considerable number of references at the end of this book.

Yet as important as carnitine, energy, and the Paleolithic diet are, the most important idea Robert presents is the need for optimal health. I hope that after you read this groundbreaking book, you will understand that carnitine, the Paleolithic Principles, the flexible menu plans, and all of the other nutritional suggestions are designed to get you health that is not merely adequate, but optimal. To the degree this book succeeds in that goal, it will change your life forever for the better.

Jeffrey Moss, D.D.S., C.N.S., C.C.N.
Hadley, Massachusetts

Note to the Reader

As a nutritionist, I have learned five things:

First, the most valuable thing you can give your cells is energy. Cells that run out of energy die before they should. This can lead to disease and premature aging. Cells that have an abundant supply of energy, however, live long and healthy lives. Because our cells run out of energy too quickly, we do not live as long as we should.

Second, our diet should incorporate the principles of the Paleolithic diet as much as possible. The Paleolithic diet is what humans ate from approximately 2.6 million years ago to 10,000 years ago. It is the single best nutrition guide we have. It is the diet our body was designed for.

Third, we will never successfully lower the rates of cancer, heart disease, and other degenerative diseases until we begin to pursue optimal—not merely adequate—health.

Fourth, for optimal health to occur, we must consume optimal levels of all beneficial nutrients, not merely the so-called essential ones. Such optimal nutrient intake is not possible from food alone. We must use supplements.

Lastly, we are all biochemically unique. Our diet and supplement plan must be tailored to meet our individual needs.

What This Book Will Show You

This book will show you how to do four things:

Energize yourself naturally

Lose body fat

Maximize brain health

Treat a range of health problems with nutrition and natural medicine

We will learn principles—not magic formulas—for health. From these principles we will learn how to make the lessons of the Paleolithic diet, the idea of optimal health, and all of the other topics of this book easy to incorporate into everyday life.

We will learn about carnitine, the premier energizing and anti-aging nutrient. Carnitine plays an important role in helping us achieve all of the above four goals. We will also look at flexible menu plans that will allow you to easily incorporate all of the principles of this book into your diet.

Choose from this book only what is useful and doable. Don't look at it as an all-or-nothing proposition. Only make dietary changes as long as they are positive and enjoyable.

Don't avoid foods because they are bad. Include foods and supplements because they are good. Start by adding quality protein, omega-3 fats, and carnitine. Continue with antioxidants, and, if possible, a more individualized diet and supplement program designed for you by a cutting-edge nutritionist. Soon you will find that the unhealthy elements of your diet will fall away with little effort.

Once your body gets a taste of health, it will only want more of it. You will find yourself addicted to something very positive: a flexible and easy way of living and eating that will put you irreversibly on the road to optimal health.

What is Carnitine?

The path to nutritional health is paved with carnitine.

—Richard Kunin, M.D.

Carnitine—the central theme of this book—is one of the nutrients that helps you turn food into energy. In that way it is similar to the B vitamins. It is remarkably similar in structure to the B vitamin choline in particular. Yet carnitine is not a true vitamin, because the body makes it in small amounts.

Carnitine is also not an amino acid, though you may hear it called that. Amino acids are building blocks that form the proteins that make up hair, nails, immune cells, and other body structures. Yet carnitine does not have an "amino group," which scientists like to see on something before they call it an amino acid. Years ago, carnitine was erroneously called an amino acid. In the common parlance it stuck—incorrectly.

So what is carnitine? It is a nutrient that does something no other nutrient can do: It acts like a forklift, picking up fats and dropping them off where the body burns them. It also plays many other roles in keeping the energy furnaces in your cells—your mitochondria—running smoothly so you can have maximal energy, health, and longevity.[1]

Acetyl-L-carnitine is a special form of carnitine that has unique protective and brain-energizing properties. We will address acetyl-L-carnitine in depth later in the book.

WHICH FOODS CONTAIN CARNITINE?

Carnitine is found predominantly in meat and animal products. Red meat is the best source. Mutton and lamb have the highest levels. Chicken and turkey also contain carnitine, though not as much as is found in red meat. Carnitine is also found to a lesser extent in milk and dairy products.

We consume about 50 mg of carnitine per day in our diet. Those who eat many servings per day of red meat get more. Strict vegetarians get little or no carnitine. Most fruits, vegetables, and grains contain almost no carnitine, with the exception of tempeh and avocados, which contain small amounts.

You can make small amounts of carnitine in your body. To do so you need the amino acids lysine and methionine; vitamins such as niacin, B_6, and vitamin C; and iron. A shortage of any of these nutrients can lower carnitine levels. Taking lysine has been found to boost carnitine levels. This is because lysine is the parent molecule from which carnitine is made. Strict vegetarians (vegans) often do not get enough lysine. Since they also consume virtually no carnitine, they have a particularly strong need to supplement with carnitine.

While we make carnitine in the body, there is substantial evidence that for optimal health we should be getting at least 250 to 500 mg in our diet daily. Humans have eaten carnitine in significant amounts for most of their history and relied on it to help keep them optimally healthy. Stone Age mankind probably ate at least 500 to 2,000 mg of carnitine per day for over 2.6 million years, and our bodies are probably used to getting that amount on a daily basis.

The real health benefits of carnitine do not come in the amount our body makes or the amount in most people's diets. We must get carnitine in optimal amounts if our goal is optimal health. And for everyone who does not want to consume large amounts of red meat—the only significant source for this nutrient—this means supplements.

THE CARNITINE ADVANTAGE

The carnitine advantage is abundant energy. Our body, as we age, experiences an energy crisis in its cells that leads to disease. Carnitine solves this problem. The energy that carnitine unleashes allows us to build health and prevent disease in a wide variety of ways.

This abundant energy that carnitine helps to deliver has made an enormous difference in the health of all my clients. It is the single most remarkable nutrient I have used in my nutrition practice over the past twelve years. No other nutrient makes my clients experience a more noticeable difference in the way they feel. They invariably report:

➤ *Improved overall well-being*
➤ *Increased weight loss*
➤ *Naturally maximized energy levels*
➤ *Lower blood cholesterol and triglyceride levels*
➤ *Reduced food cravings*
➤ *Increased energy during exercise and better exercise endurance*
➤ *Increased heart health and a reduced need for heart medications*
➤ *Better circulation*
➤ *Relief from depression*
➤ *Optimized brain energy*

My favorite thing about carnitine is it's ability to increase overall well-being. This tells me that carnitine is working on a very basic level to increase overall body health.

Why is carnitine's effect so profound? Because it is so basic. It is like a wheel on your car. If you are driving with only three wheels, and the fourth wheel bearing is scraping on the ground, you will not go far. If I tell you that something as simple as another wheel can get you going, give you more speed, deliver better handling, and give you a smoother ride, you may not believe that one thing can do all this—but it can. It is because you are missing something so basic that you stand to enjoy so many benefits. Carnitine is just that basic and profound in its effects on the body.

The invention of money by the Sumerians thousands of years ago was the catalyst that allowed for the growth of modern societies. Why? Money is pure societal potential. It can be turned into anything—streets, highways, buildings, bridges, labor to create and service a city—whatever is needed for the growth and health of a complex society. So basic an invention as money seems obvious, but it was a great innovation. It allowed things to happen that otherwise would never have been possible because it allowed for a universal currency that could be used to accomplish any goal. The optimal energy carnitine provides is the cellular equivalent of money.

Carnitine and the energy it creates is just as profound and far-reaching. If you give your cells the ability to make optimal levels of energy, they can use it to do whatever they want: build and renew cell membranes, create and maintain cell structures, and replicate and protect cell information. In short, they can use it to make themselves work better and last longer.

Remember when your aunt Edna gave you that fruitcake for the holidays? You wished she had given you the twenty dollars she spent on it instead. This does not make you materialistic. You just want that which suits your needs—there is nothing wrong with that. You sat there looking at that fruitcake thinking of the millions of things you could have done with that twenty bucks. It's a normal reaction.

Our cells also know best what they need. When we give our cells carnitine and increase their energy, they take that energy and do what they want with it. They use it to create a better defense against viruses and bacteria, to protect and regenerate their cell membranes, or to rejuvenate themselves in any way they desire. And isn't it best to let the cells of our body decide what they need?

This is what natural medicine is: letting the body decide what it wants, not forcing it to accept something it does not want. Cells look at drugs like unwanted fruitcakes. They grudgingly consume them to make you happy, and often as a result get sick. Cells usually want nutrients, not misguided drug therapy. Most doctors are as in touch with the real needs of the body as Aunt Edna is with your wants and desires. Drugs can be useful, but they are far from the perfect metabolic gift.

This is what carnitine and all the other nutrients that promote the structure and function of your body are: the perfect metabolic gift. You can give your body nothing better than that which it is made out of—carnitine and all of the other healing nutrients. It makes sense to use first what the body is made out of. This is the best way to heal.

You hopefully now realize that the most important healing element in your body is energy. Therefore, the most important healing nutrients are those that promote optimal energy levels. Cells with abundant energy are free of disease. Make your cells energetic and you will increase your chances of living a long life. The best nutrient to help you do this is carnitine.

Everyone Who Wants to Lose Weight Should Take Carnitine

Carnitine is the best nutrient there is for promoting weight loss. My clients have taught me this. Scientific research has shown me this as well. When you see how carnitine works in the body, you will understand why.

Carnitine is the gatekeeper for fat-burning. It picks up fat and puts it into the part of the cell that burns it off. Every human being that has ever walked the planet has had carnitine as a natural part of his or her metabolism to burn fat.

Limited carnitine, limited fat-burning. Optimal carnitine, optimal fat burning. It's that simple. Carnitine is the most important nutrient for naturally supporting the weight loss process, and the results you can get if you take it in the right doses (1,000 mg and beyond) can be quite dramatic.

CARNITINE CASE HISTORY

Tina is a seventy-seven-year-old type II diabetic who got unusually stunning results from carnitine. By taking 1,000 mg of carnitine per day, she lost 30 pounds, dropping from 183 to 153 pounds, in a little over three months. All of this happened simply by taking carnitine. She was so thrilled with the results that she has all her friends taking carnitine. She has now maintained her weight loss for six months.

Why do we have weight-loss drugs when carnitine is freely available? Obesity is not a drug deficiency. But it is almost always a functional carnitine deficiency.

WHAT IS A FUNCTIONAL DEFICIENCY?

A functional deficiency of a nutrient is an intake of a nutrient lower than the amount needed to promote optimal health. Functional deficiency is a much more advanced way of looking at nutrient needs. You may have enough vitamin C to avoid its deficiency disease scurvy, but if you do not have enough C to prevent colds, reduce risk of heart disease and neutralize carcinogens, you have a functional deficiency of vitamin C. When it comes to nutrients, merely avoiding deficiency diseases is passé, because the amount that prevents deficiency will not promote optimal health.

Let's think of it in terms of money. You could survive on ten thousand dollars a year, but you could live more fully and freely on $100,000 annually. You would have a functional deficiency of money at the lower level. Your essentials would be met, but optimal living—from an economic standpoint—would elude you. You would not have an outright deficiency of money, but you would be far from having enough to enjoy life to the fullest.

So it is with nutrients. Americans are marginal in their consumption of folic acid, vitamin E, magnesium, zinc, chromium, and selenium, and for other nutrients we barely consume enough to cover our basic needs. But even when we eat a very healthy diet, the amount of nutrients in food does not promote optimal health and longevity. The real benefits of nutrients come at the optimal level of intake. If we really want to thrive, stay slim, and be healthy, then we will have to look at more than what food supplies, and look beyond merely avoiding deficiency.

So when it comes to promoting weight loss, we must make sure that we have optimal—not merely adequate—levels of carnitine.

CARNITINE SHOULD BE THE #1 WEIGHT LOSS DRUG

Why is carnitine not yet used by everyone who wants to lose weight? Perhaps because drug companies do not have enough economic incentive to research and market it. Drug companies make money on drugs they research, patent, and collect royalties on. The process requires more than three hundred million dollars. Carnitine is available over the counter at health food stores at prices drug companies cannot compete with. They would never recoup such a sizeable investment if they researched and promoted carnitine, so they don't.

Carnitine would also be much more widely used if people knew how to use it. You need to take at least 1,000 mg per day to help promote weight loss, according to my clinical experience. Sometimes people will use a weight loss formula that has 50 mg of carnitine in it. For promoting weight loss and energy this is a meaningless dose. People often use these low doses without results. They then think that carnitine does not help promote weight loss. This is like throwing a glass of water on a burning building and concluding that water does not put out fires. You don't know the effectiveness of a compound until you use the right dose. And for optimally promoting weight loss, the right dose of carnitine is sometimes as high as 4 grams (4,000 mg) per day.

My clinical experience has also taught me that carnitine works best with a diet that is low in carbohydrates (sugars and starches). At most, carbohydrates should comprise no more than 50 percent of the total calories consumed for carnitine to work optimally. This is because a higher intake of carbohydrates can promote an elevated level of the hormone insulin, which inhibits optimal carnitine activity. Also, eating a diet rich in omega-3 fats improves carnitine's performance.

OMEGA-3 FATS

Omega-3 fats are health-promoting fats found in a reddish-brown seed known as the flaxseed, as well as the oil made from it, flaxseed oil. Omega-3s are also abundant in cold-water fish such as salmon, sardines, mackerel, and tuna, and are found in trace amounts in green leafy vegetables. These fats are one of the most important nutrients in our diet for preventing heart disease, cancer, obesity, depression, and inflammatory conditions. Most Americans do not eat enough of these fats.

Carnitine also works best when the carnitine tartrate form is used. This is the most effective and stable form of carnitine for use in supplements, and I urge you to look for it if you want the best results. I have found that other forms will often work, but not as reliably as the tartrate. This is probably due to the extraordinary purity of carnitine tartrate. Impurities found in other forms can interfere with the action of carnitine.

If you do not experience any results with a carnitine supplement, you should try another brand, and make sure it uses the tartrate form. Carnitine tartrate has a tart taste, so when you open a capsule of it, you should be able to taste a certain tartness. Otherwise, you do not have the real thing.

WEIGHT LOSS IS MULTIFACTORIAL

You need more than carnitine to lose weight successfully. You need a diet with optimal amounts of protein and omega-3 fats, rich in essential nutrients, and low in carbohydrates. Exercise is also very helpful. But the most important thing that you need to lose weight is something many of us lack: emotional and spiritual wellness.

Food is a very emotional issue. There are many depressed people in this country who overeat to cover pain. There are many people who do not love themselves and therefore do not feel they deserve health and do not pursue it. And there are those who are so spiritually asleep that they are somehow not connected enough with their body to know they need to take care of it. There are also, unfortunately, many people who have had unpleasant experiences as children—physical and verbal violations—that make them reluctant to be attractive. For them, extra weight is a protective shield. It insulates them emotionally and prevents them from being involved on a level where there is still a lot of pain.

Most of the overweight people I have counseled have psychological issues that must be dealt with. Otherwise they will not love themselves enough to want health and happiness. This is particularly true for those who are a hundred pounds or more overweight. For such people, emotional and spiritual solutions are needed first, not a diet or supplements. Then health and happiness and an attractive physique can come into being when the right nutritional strategy is added. For reasons I do not know, those who weigh three hundred or more pounds rarely keep their weight off. This has been my experience, and perhaps highlights the shortcoming of my only being a nutritionist and trying to manage the grossly obese. I can only help people on a certain level—when they are emotionally ready to make positive changes.

So forgive me at times if I make weight loss or the attainment of optimal health sound like a simple biochemical thing. It is not. You have to want it to happen. You have to be prepared for happiness emotionally and spiritually, which many people are not. There are changes that will happen in your life when you become optimally healthy that you must be ready for on every level or they will not endure, if they happen at all.

I am excited because I have seen these positive changes happen many times, and I know that optimal health is attainable. But realize that there are many kinds of wellness beyond the narrow scope of nutrition—the focus of this book—that you must pursue to get there.

So, if you have wellness on the psychological and spiritual levels and are now ready to complete the picture with wellness on the physical level, this book is for you. Good luck, and I hope you enjoy every step of the way on your path to optimal wellness!

Top Ten Kinds of People Most Likely to Benefit from Carnitine

❶ *Those who need more energy!* Those who are always tired should first rule out thyroid problems, hemochromatosis, or other medical problems that can cause fatigue. But carnitine can always be useful for anyone who needs more energy.

❷ *Those who want to lose weight.* Combined with a low carbohydrate diet, carnitine is the most effective nutrient there is for promoting weight loss.

❸ *Those who want to promote heart health.* Carnitine is crucial for heart health, and combined with CoQ10, vitamin E, magnesium, and herbs like cactus and hawthorn, carnitine heads up a list of key heart-health promoters.

❹ *Athletes.* Carnitine promotes maximum endurance and peak performance in aerobic sports.

❺ *Those who want optimal immune function.* Carnitine energizes the cells of the immune system, thereby making them better able to protect you. Carnitine also increases the number of protective white blood cells.

❻ *Lactating women and infants.* Carnitine is an absolutely essential nutrient for babies to get, either through breastmilk or formula.

❼ *Vegetarians of all ages, especially those who consume no animal products of any kind.* Since animal products are the only foods that contain appreciable amounts of carnitine, strict vegetarians have a special need to take carnitine supplements for optimal health.

❽ *Those who want maximal brain health and who want to do everything they can to prevent the loss of brain function throughout their life.* Acetyl-L-carnitine is one of the most important brain-longevity nutrients we have.

❾ *Those who are under stress.* Carnitine and acetyl-L-carnitine are very helpful at protecting the body from the damaging effects of stress, which, unchecked, can accelerate the aging process.

❿ *Those with a range of other ailments, including male infertility, cancer, AIDS, chronic fatigue, fibromyalgia, and liver problems.*[2]

Carnitine Slows the Aging Process

The main reason to take carnitine on a regular basis is that it is one of the most important nutrients for slowing the aging process. Energy is the greatest antiaging force there is. The more energy your cells have, the slower they age. Because body levels of carnitine—our premier energizing nutrient—decline as we get older, cells are not as energetic as we age.[3] This decreased level of cellular energy is one of the reasons we see the aging process actually accelerate as we get older. Carnitine and acetyl-L-carnitine do much to help slow down aging throughout life, and are especially important as we age.

Why is energy antiaging? It is energy in our cells that repairs them and keeps them healthy. Ideally, all energizing nutrients should be used in a balance for this antiaging effect, but carnitine and acetyl-L-carnitine are two of the most important.

Carnitine also prevents cells from self-destructing when faced with environmental toxins like free radicals.[4] Free radicals are compounds made by our body and found in our foods and environment that damage and destroy cells. They are implicated in causing a wide range of diseases. As we age, our body is less able to protect itself from free radicals. Carnitine and acetyl-L-carnitine powerfully protect us from them.[5]

Carnitine also keeps the immune system strong, especially as we age.[6] This is very important, for our immune system gets weaker as life goes on, and we are more susceptible to life-threatening bouts of pneumonia, the flu, and other infectious diseases.

Carnitine and acetyl-L-carnitine also help to create a healthier balance of fats in the blood and the cells of the body. This in turn helps prevent heart disease and also reduces the likelihood of diseases associated with inflammation.[7]

Carnitine also protects our cells against the forces of poor circulation and low oxygen levels. As we age, we usually have poorer circulation. This allows cells less oxygen to live on, and often causes us to age more quickly. The reason? When we have less oxygen, we make less energy in cells and they can die. Carnitine protects against this, and allows our cells to thrive in environments of lower oxygen concentration.[8] Indeed, as we grow older, and our circulation declines, carnitine requirements greatly increase. We need more in order to protect our cells from the damage that can occur due to a lack of optimal oxygen levels in tissues.

Carnitine is an important longevity nutrient for the heart. It is one of the most important compounds for the prevention of a range of ailments that affect the heart and circulatory system. Carnitine simply helps the heart work better, especially as we age. It also helps treat many ailments associated with the aging heart, such as angina, congestive heart failure, and the damage to the heart that occurs with heart attacks.

So, how much carnitine do we need? Traditionally, nutritionists have said that we need only enough to avoid deficiency diseases. But aging too quickly, heart disease, and Alzheimer's may really be long-term functional carnitine deficiencies. We need enough carnitine to avoid these ailments and to give our body the optimal health it deserves.

If you are flying from Los Angeles to New York and your flight plan is off by just a few degrees, you will end up in Boston. So it is with health. Getting the right amount of carnitine throughout life—along with all the minerals, vitamins, and all the other health-promoting nutrients we need—is essential to prevent disease. We have to decide early on in our flight of life what we need nutritionally if we hope to arrive at our destination of vital health toward the end. The best way to get there is to set our course on the path of optimal wellness as early as possible.

So what should be our optimal intake of essential nutrients, and carnitine in particular? To help answer that, let's look at the Paleolithic diet. This is the diet humans ate from 2.6 million years ago up until the advent of agriculture 10,000 years ago. This is the diet that we thrived on for most of our history. It is the one our body is designed for. It is the best nutrition teacher we have.

So let us now take a short detour away from carnitine as we look at the principles of healthy eating from the Paleolithic perspective. This will give us an important background from which we will develop the Carnitine Program—an eating program designed to create optimal health and help us get the greatest possible benefits from taking carnitine.

Stone Age Nutrition

Progress, far from consisting in change, depends on retentiveness.

—George Santayana

Virtually all chronic disease results from abandoning the Paleolithic diet.

—Leigh Broadhurst, Ph.D.

The terms "Paleolithic," "Stone Age," and "hunter-gatherer" are interchangeable, and refer to the period from 2.6 million years ago until the advent of farming, approximately 10,000 years ago. Paleolithic, or Stone Age, nutrition is the study of what humans ate during this period. Looking at this large expanse of human nutrition can teach us a lot about what our bodies have adapted to, for our bodies have not changed genetically in any meaningful way since we left our hunter-gatherer lifestyle.

The Stone Age diet consisted of meat from every kind of animal, including organ meats and brain. Insects, worms, nuts and seeds, and occasionally eggs were eaten. Wild plants and fruits were eaten, but not in the northern latitudes, and not in the winter in temperate zones. No grains, no dairy products, no lentils or beans were eaten. The Paleolithic diet is what you would eat if you were dropped off in a forest, African savannah, or colder climates with only those tools and weapons you could make by hand.

Then, somewhere from ten thousand to five thousand years ago, farming began, and three new elements entered our diet:

> Grain products (barley, then wheat and spelt, and later corn and the bread products made from them)
> Dairy products (cow's milk, cheese, yogurt, and butter)
> Dried legumes such as soybeans, peanuts, and pinto beans. Prior to this, legumes were eaten rarely and almost always in the green state, for example, green peas.

These foods gradually began to replace meat, which was now becoming more difficult to obtain. The shortage of large game animals is what researchers believe drove us into farming—a move we made reluctantly. Originating in Turkey, wheat and other grains slowly spread throughout the world, becoming the nutritional fad that caught on forever. Grains allowed humans to get the calories and other nutrients they needed to survive the meat shortage. They created an abundant food supply that promoted the growth in population that would allow us to populate every part of the planet.

The use of grains as the centerpiece of the diet had bad effects. This switch away from meat saw humans lose six inches in height, suffer a dramatic increase in tooth decay and bone malformations, suffer increased infant mortality, and acquire many diseases not known in hunter-gatherer groups such as adult onset diabetes and coronary heart disease. The move from meat to grains allowed for more people. But the people who ate grains were much less robust than the meat-eaters who preceded them.[9]

THE PALEOLITHIC FOOD PYRAMID

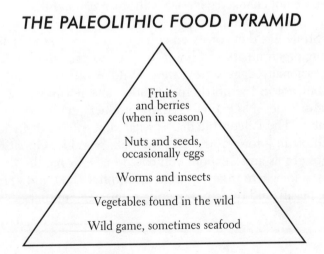

Fruits
and berries
(when in season)

Nuts and seeds,
occasionally eggs

Worms and insects

Vegetables found in the wild

Wild game, sometimes seafood

Pretty sparse-looking pyramid, isn't it? But that is what humans existed on for most of history. We may do best on exactly this regime. These are exactly the kinds of fuel our body is designed for. And notice that there are no ratios: the relative amounts of any food depend on what was available in each area during each season. The pyramid structure around this diet is only used to compare it to our food pyramid. There is no evidence from the study of human history or nutrition that a pyramid is a good template for diet design. There are groups that eat 60 percent of their calories from fat and thrive (the Inuit), while some eat less fat and do just as well. Fats in their natural state in wild foods eaten in the context of a nutrient-rich diet have never caused disease. As we shall see, principles are more useful than formulas for understanding health.

PALEONUTRIENTS

The Paleolithic intake of vitamins and minerals was much higher than what our government recommends we eat today. According to the most recent estimates,[10] Paleolithic mankind ate:

Nutrient	Paleolithic Intake	RDA	Current U.S. Intake
Vitamin C	604 mg	60 mg	77–109 mg
Vitamin E	33 mg	8–10 mg	7–10 mg
Calcium	1,956 mg	800–1200 mg	750 mg
Magnesium	700 mg	350 mg	250 mg
Potassium	10,500 mg	3,500 mg	2,500 mg
Zinc	43 mg	12–15 mg	5–14 mg
Fiber	50–104 grams	25–35 grams*	10 grams

*Amount recommended by the American Dietetic Association

Paleolithic mankind got more of every nutrient than we do, sometimes manyfold more.

PALEOCARBS AND NEOCARBS: AN IMPORTANT DISTINCTION

Carbohydrates are the sugars, simple and complex, found in foods like fruits, vegetables, tubers, grains, breads, pasta, rolls, cookies, cakes, candies, juices, and soda.

Carbohydrates come in two varieties: paleocarbs, the kind we have eaten throughout our history, and neocarbs, those grain- and legume-based and refined carbohydrates that have surfaced in recent history.

Paleocarbs (good)

Paleocarbs include vegetables, fruits, and perhaps tubers. Paleolithic fruits were not eaten throughout the year except in the tropics and were smaller and less sweet than those eaten today.

Neocarbs (tolerable to bad)

Neocarbs include grains and legumes, especially the flour products, which did not exist for most of human history. The worst of the neocarbs include sugar and white-flour products, which offer the body little nutrition.

Although everyone considers whole grains a virtuous food, this is not always the case. Excessive consumption of whole grains, particularly wheat, can cause problems. Phytates are present in such foods as whole wheat bread. During the second World War, whole-wheat bread became much more widely consumed, and the phytate content of this bread greatly decreased calcium and magnesium absorption in those who ate it.[11] This switch to wholemeal bread caused rickets in children who ate significant quantities of it. Those who are fond of eating whole-wheat regularly should take extra calcium and magnesium to counter the mineral-binding effects of phytates.

Fiber has its place in our diet, but we should opt more toward soluble fibers that do not have this mineral-blocking effect. Soluble fibers are found in flaxmeal, oatmeal, psyllium seeds, fruits, and vegetables. Oats in general are a much better grain for you than wheat because they are much lower in gluten, which many people are sensitive to. While fiber from fruits and vegetables appears to be cancer-preventive, it is not clear whether fiber from grains has this effect.[12]

WE ALL REACT DIFFERENTLY TO GRAINS

This Paleolithic discussion should not lead us to conclude that no one should ever eat grains. The human race is now dependent on grains for its survival. We just need to appreciate that some can tolerate them better than others, and that more grain is not always better. Just remember: they're new, and many of us may do better to avoid them completely.

UBIQUIFOODS

In Paleolithic times, virtually all of our carbohydrates came from paleocarbs: that is, fruits and vegetables. Today in America, less than one fourth of the carbohydrates we eat come from these foods. Most of the rest come from grain, grain products, and sugars. The worst part about the carbohydrate story is the creation of what I call "ubiquifoods." These are foods that are nearly omnipresent in our diet to the point of causing nutritional and immunological insult. Examples of ubiquifoods include wheat, corn, dairy products, and soybeans. These are foods that all of us eat nearly every day because they are incorporated into many different processed foods. Wheat is a good example. We can eat wheat cereal or a muffin made from wheat for breakfast, a sandwich on wheat bread for lunch, and a dinner with wheat rolls or pasta. We snack on crackers, donuts, and other wheat-based foods. The body was never meant to eat the same food over and over like this, particularly a grain that is so new to our physiology. But this is what happens, thanks to the malleability of ubiquifoods and the wizardry of food processors. The result is food allergies, autoimmune diseases, and a lack of nutritional variation that can cause nutrient imbalances and deficiencies. Such ubiquifoods were never present in the Paleolithic diet, and a much greater variation of food sources exists in the wild. We must follow our ancestors' example and eat a widely varied diet if our goal is optimal health.

We will soon look at the Paleolithic principles. They are the best way of understanding and incorporating the lessons of Paleolithic nutrition into our everyday lives. Because there are so many different ways of eating in the wild, depending on where in the world you are, there is no single "Paleolithic Diet" we can arrive at. But there are principles we can derive from the way our ancestors ate that we can use to help us intelligently hunt for food as we walk down the danger-filled aisles of the supermarket.

But before we look at these Paleolithic principles, let's look at the shortcomings of our own government's food pyramid. Its misguided notions of nutrition do nothing to incorporate the powerful lessons of Paleolithic nutrition.

Top Ten Problems with the Food Pyramid

Teach principles, not formulas

—Richard Feynman

The food pyramid has great influence. It is the nutritional compass our government created to direct our nation to health. It is not working. The reason? It is in direct opposition to the diet we ate for most of human existence.

THE USDA FOOD GUIDE PYRAMID

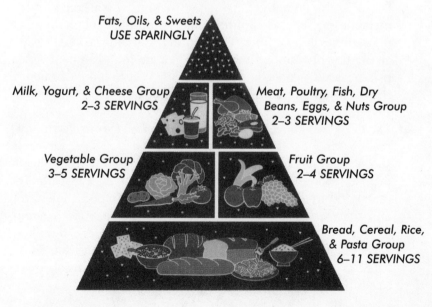

Fats, Oils, & Sweets
USE SPARINGLY

Milk, Yogurt, & Cheese Group
2–3 SERVINGS

Meat, Poultry, Fish, Dry
Beans, Eggs, & Nuts Group
2–3 SERVINGS

Vegetable Group
3–5 SERVINGS

Fruit Group
2–4 SERVINGS

Bread, Cereal, Rice,
& Pasta Group
6–11 SERVINGS

The food pyramid was built to help people understand basic nutrition. In that sense it may be considered a lit matchstick in the dark. It is better than nothing. It does recommend eating more vegetables, which is a good idea. The food pyramid may help illuminate some basic ideas about healthy eating, but it is far from the blazing torch we need to lead us to optimal health. This is in part due to the fact that the food pyramid was actually redesigned after food manufacturers saw it and had their input. This kind of influence makes about as much sense as asking prisoners for input on a new penal code.

The food pyramid, therefore, is a marriage of lobbying and a nutritional stance that does not recognize the importance of Paleolithic nutrition, omega-3 fatty acids, and the healthy-eating principles we shall outline below. That is why it is such a failure. It is hardly the ideal diet for our Paleolithic bodies.

Here are the top ten problems with the food pyramid, and some suggested solutions:

❶ *The food pyramid says to eat fats sparingly.* This is not the answer to our fat-related disease problems such as heart disease and cancer. The number one nutrition problem-causing disease in America is omega-3 fatty acid deficiency. We are not eating too much fat. We are eating the wrong kinds and missing the good fats. We also do not get enough of the nutrients needed for fat metabolism, such as carnitine, and an optimal supply of vitamins, minerals, and fiber. The solution? Put omega-3 fatty acids at the top of the food pyramid. They are found in cold-water fish, flaxseed, canola, and soybean oils. We should recommend the inclusion of quality fats, not fat avoidance.

❷ *The food pyramid recommends that everyone eat six to eleven servings of starch per day.* This is wrong for many people. Research shows that diets high in carbohydrates increase the risk of heart disease among many people, and that a diet high in carbohydrates (60 to 70 percent or more) can upset blood cholesterol and triglyceride levels. Many people are also allergic to grain products. Our Stone Age ancestors ate no grains for 2.6 million years, the vast majority of our history. Grain servings should be listed as zero to five per day, with the rest of the carbohydrate needs being made up by starchy vegetables.

❸ *The food pyramid does not allow for the fact that grains contain many antinutrients* like phytates, which block nutrient absorption. Phytates block mineral absorption, especially calcium, iron, and zinc, three minerals that are often deficient in the American diet. Grains also contain a compound called pyridoxine glucoside which can block vitamin B_6 absorption by up to 80 percent. Grains also contain factors that can promote rickets, and other compounds that promote inflammation. And as nutrition researcher Loren Cordain, Ph.D., has pointed out, the major deficiency diseases—scurvy, beriberi, pellagra, and others—have occurred mainly in cultures that eat a lot of grains. This is not to say that no one should eat grains. But there are many questions as to whether we should be emphasizing a grain-based diet for everyone. So, zero to five servings per day would be a more ideal universal recommendation for grain products.

❹ *The food pyramid makes no distinction regarding the kind of carbohydrates people should eat.* Refined white bread and a sweet potato both satisfy the food pyramid, while the latter is infinitely more health-promoting. The carbohydrate section of the food pyramid should insist on "avoiding refined carbohydrates such as white flour and sugar as much as possible."

❺ *A pyramid is not a good template for diet recommendations.* We all need different ratios of fat to protein to carbohydrates, and these varying ratios are difficult to fit into a pyramid. Some thrive on a 30 percent fat diet while others need more. There are also those who should eat equal amounts of all three macronutrients: fats, proteins, and carbohydrates. So some will need a food rectangle and some a food rhombus. Others will have such fluctuating needs day to day that they will need a food amoeba!

❻ *The food pyramid does not adequately suggest the need to vary foods.* We must change our foods daily and with the seasons to help prevent food allergies and to maximize the nutritional value of our diet. We should eat more fruit in the summer, less fruit and more starchy vegetables in the winter, and rotate our sources of protein throughout the year.

❼ *The food pyramid has inadequate protein recommendations,* especially for those who exercise or are under stress. Higher protein intake also raises beneficial HDL cholesterol and is heart-protective. The range of protein intake must be made much greater.

❽ *The animal products recommended in the food pyramid should be from animals fed grasses, not grains.* This would help Americans get more omega-3 fats which are found in grass- but not grain-fed animals. Increased intake of omega-3 fats would help us prevent many diseases, especially heart disease.

❾ *The food pyramid recommends that everyone eat dairy products,* which some do not tolerate at all. Those with dairy allergies, such as children with recurrent ear infections, should eat no dairy products. Dairy is not a food that everyone should eat. Though rich in calcium, dairy products are not the only foods that supply it. Greens, sesame seeds, and all nuts and seeds contain calcium and other bone-building nutrients.

❿ *The biggest problem with the food pyramid is that it does not allow for biochemical individuality.* There is no one diet for everyone and there is no one formula of recommendations that will work for everyone. A much wider latitude of eating possibilities must be built into the food pyramid if it is to help everyone attain optimal health.

The biggest reason for the failure of the food pyramid is not merely its mistaken love of grains and lack of key information, but also the fact that it attempts to teach health with a formula. What we need are principles. Only principles can be easily worked into the fluidity of our lives and address our individual needs.

If the right nutrition principles were taught to and implemented by Americans, we would be much healthier. And the principles that would help us the most are those that are based on what we have eaten and thrived on for most of our history: Paleolithic principles.

The Paleolithic Principles of Healthy Eating

All humans require similar ranges of both macro and micronutrients and all human groups have similar anatomical, physiological, and endocrine functions in regard to diet and nutrition. We were all hunter-gatherers dependent upon wild plants and animals, and these dietary selective pressures shaped our present-day nutritional requirements.

—Loren Cordain, Ph.D.

A revolution means going all the way back around to where you started from.

—Igor Stravinsky

Here are the ten Paleolithic principles of healthy eating. Follow them as best you can. The more my clients follow these principles, the healthier they are. They should, however, be adapted to individual needs. Some will do fine with small amounts of grains while others will feel best when they avoid them completely. Some tolerate dairy products, while many people feel better when they avoid them or switch to goat's milk. Vegetarians may not eat animal products but can benefit from the other principles. Use these principles in whatever way suits you best.

❶ *Eat high-quality animal products if this does not conflict with your religious or animal-rights convictions.* Ideally this should be wild game, other lean meat, or seafood. Meat has been consumed by mankind throughout our history and is health-promoting as long as it is from animals that are allowed to live in the wild or are fed a diet that reflects their natural eating patterns. In other words, animals should be fed grasses and flaxseeds, not merely grains. Lean meat raises HDL cholesterol, lowers triglycerides, and protects against heart disease, the main killer in our country.

❷ *Eat a diet balanced in fat quality.* Notice that I do not recommend a low-fat diet. What is more important is that the fat you eat be balanced between omega-3, omega-6, and saturated fats, all of which benefit the body when eaten in the right ratios to each other. Avoid toxic fats like margarine and mass-market refined vegetable oils. The polyunsaturated craze that has caused Americans to overeat refined safflower, sunflower, and corn oils has caused more health problems than it has solved.

❸ *Food should be eaten, when possible, in its whole state.* There is always more nutrition in whole food than a fraction taken from it. Freshly ground flaxseeds offer more health benefits than flaxseed oil, though flaxseed oil is still very health-promoting. Never trim away the healthy fats from salmon. Fruits are much better for you than fruit juices.

❹ *Cook foods minimally.* I am not, however, recommending you eat an all-raw-food diet. Meat should never be eaten raw, though our Stone Age ancestors ate it this way. Meat should just not be overcooked. It should never be blackened as is done in Cajun cooking. Blackening foods creates a range of toxic compounds that stress the body. Meat should be eaten well-done, however, in this age of E. coli, salmonella, and other heat-sensitive pathogens. Vegetables should be raw or steamed, never boiled. There are those who do better on more cooked foods, and in the winter, eating too many raw foods can be inappropriate and make you feel cold. Strike the balance between raw and cooked foods that works best for you.

❺ *Grain and dairy products are foods that are relatively new to humanity.* Some tolerate them better than others. When grains compose more than 50 percent of the diet, they have been documented to cause health problems such as mineral deficiencies.[13] This should be kept in mind when designing a diet. We cannot blindly call grain and dairy products health-promoting for everyone. For many people, they are not. Those who do tolerate small amounts of these foods often do not do well on large amounts. As Dr. Loren Cordain says, "Just because a small amount of grain products may be good for you does not mean a lot will be better." It may be worse.

6 *Large amounts of fat and carbohydrates should not be eaten together.* This was never done by Stone Age man. Diets that have high amounts of fat, as is the case with the traditional Eskimo diet, are also low in carbohydrates, while the diets of equatorial peoples that are higher in carbohydrates are usually lower in fats. The combination of high-carbohydrate and high-fat intake is new to mankind and is disease-causing. It is not a diet available in the wild. So do not think that high-fat diets cause disease. They do not, unless they are combined with a high intake of carbohydrates.

7 *Eat organic foods as often as possible.* Organic foods are those grown without pesticides, herbicides, or fungicides. Many of these compounds are carcinogenic and toxic to the nervous system when eaten throughout life. Most of them are not adequately tested for their effects on humans. More and more farmers are switching to organic farming methods, so the price of organic produce should continue to come down.

8 *Eat foods that are grown locally and that therefore reflect the seasonal changes of your surroundings.* Winter in northern climates is a time for less fruit and more root vegetables. A higher fat intake is also appropriate in the winter, especially of omega-3 fats found in flaxseeds and cold-water fish. Eating according to the seasons also allows us to rotate foods naturally and get more variety and a more balanced nutrient intake. Such varied food intake also helps protect us from food allergies that can come from eating the same foods throughout the year. We should trust that nature will supply foods at different seasons that are in accordance with our needs.

❾ *We should eat as great a variety of foods as possible at all times.* Paleolithic mankind ate many different kinds of meat, vegetables, fruits, nuts, and seeds. Our diet is overly based on foods such as wheat, dairy, corn, and soy—foods I call ubiquifoods— foods we eat too often and in too great a quantity because they are processed into so many different convenience foods. Beyond the fact that the above-mentioned foods are not true paleofoods, their sheer monotony does not give us exposure to all the nutrients we need for optimal health. Variety is one of the most important principles of nutrition and especially paleonutrition. Eating a wide variety of foods is also very enjoyable!

❿ *Eat according to the needs of your ancestors.* Hispanics, for example, may need to limit their intake of carbohydrates, particularly sugar and refined-grain products. These foods may predispose them to diseases related to high insulin levels, such as obesity, type II diabetes, and heart disease. If you come from a people group that herded animals for thousands of years, you may tolerate dairy products better than others. Those of Mediterranean ancestry may be best suited to the Mediterranean diet that is being suggested (wrongly) for everyone. We need to modify the Paleolithic principles to meet our individual needs and those that our ancestry suggests.

The Problems with a Vegetarian Diet

Twenty-two years of tofu is a lot of time.

> —Paul Obis, founder of *Vegetarian Times*, on why he started eating meat again[14]

The most damaging concept to our health today is that we would all be better off if we were vegetarians. And with this usually comes the assertion that humans are somehow designed to be vegetarians. All of this is fallacious.

If we are designed to eat anything, it is animal products along with uncultivated fruits and vegetables. Research suggests that hunter-gatherer populations got 56 percent of their calories from animal productsand thrived.[15] For the vast majority of our history we never ate grains, and the recent introduction of grain products has caused more problems than it has solved.

You can eat a vegetarian diet and be healthy. And there are those who seem to do fine on a high-carbohydrate diet high in grains, though they rarely look robust and energetic when they walk in my office. This is because it is a lot harder to achieve optimal health as a vegetarian. You are more likely to be pulled down the path of too many carbohydrates and not enough protein. Worst of all, you are eating a diet your body was not designed for. You are an omnivore, no matter what your favorite columnist in your health magazine says. You have to realize that limiting yourself to one part of the food spectrum limits your health.

The criticisms one hears of meat-based diets are correct. We need to increase the quality of animal products. We need to stop animal abuse. We need to stop drugging animals with antibiotics and hormones. We need to start feeding animals grasses, flaxseeds, and other things that will increase the omega-3 content of meat and eggs. But saying that we should eat no animal products is wrong. It is people abuse. It weakens our health and denies us the diet we were designed to eat: one that features meat as well as vegetables.

I have seen many people become vegetarians—including myself—and not been pleased by the results. Health and vitality decline. I respect those who love animals or who for spiritual reasons do not want to eat meat. I listen attentively to those who claim that a vegetarian diet may help those with certain types of cancer. They may be right. But for most of us, vegetarianism does not improve our health. We ate meat for 2.6 million years and were very healthy. When we were forced to become farmers due to the shortage of game animals, our health declined.

A healthy vegetarian diet is far better than the junk-food laden standard American diet. But it still pales when compared to the health-promoting power of a diet built on Paleolithic principles. If our development as humans depended on the presence of meat in our diet, it is illogical to now conclude that an optimal diet must somehow exclude it.

The word "meat" is part of the problem. The Eskimos have forty-four words for ice. We need forty-four words for meat. Junky meats like bologna cannot compare with the health-promoting power of wild game or even the flank steak in your supermarket. Calling them all meat is confusing. We need a new language to fully understand the many beneficial properties of the health-promoting end of the meat spectrum.

Vegetarianism's benefits are the benefits of getting half of the Paleolithic picture right: eating lots of vegetables, as well as avoiding junky meat products. Vegetarians get more antioxidants like vitamin C and carotenoids through their diet. This is good. But this does not come from eating less meat. It comes from eating more vegetables. And eating more vegetables is not something only vegetarians can do. Meat-eaters should eat more vegetables as well, while also incorporating more health-promoting fresh meat products. Vegetarians, through their blanket condemnation of meat, are in essence practicing foodism: they reject all meat because some of it—bologna, high-fat meats, and aged meat—is health-impairing.

Remember, you can be a vegetarian and be healthy. It is just a lot more work.

Here, then, are the top ten problems with the vegetarian diet:

❶ *The vegetarian diet is high in carbohydrates.* High-carbohydrate diets increase the risk of heart disease by upsetting insulin metabolism and raising the blood levels of triglycerides.[16] One review found that female vegetarians have a higher rate of coronary heart disease deaths than female meat-eaters.[17]

❷ A *strict vegetarian diet is devoid of carnitine and low in its nutritional precursor, lysine.* Vegetarian diets are also low in the antioxidant and immune-boosting nutrient taurine and low in the valuable omega-3 fatty acids EPA and DHA.

❸ A *diet high in grains antagonizes the activity of the B vitamin biotin.* Biotin is essential for healthy fat metabolism.[18]

❹ *The vegetarian diet is high in carbohydrates and often high in sugars as well,* and this can increase the likelihood of a yeast overgrowth and other forms of dysbiosis. Such bowel overgrowths of undesirable fungi and bacteria have been associated with a range of health problems including neurological disorders.[19]

❺ *Diets high in carbohydrates and low in protein increase food cravings,* particularly for more carbohydrates.[20] This can lead to carbohydrate overeating, blood sugar imbalances, and eventually, adrenal exhaustion and burnout.

❻ *Diets high in bread and cereal products are associated with an increased risk of breast*[21] *and colorectal cancer.*[22]

❼ *Diets high in grains are associated with an excess of omega-6 fats and a shortage of omega-3 fats.* This excessive consumption of omega-6 fats increases the risk of heart disease and other inflammatory disorders.[23]

❽ *Vegetarians have a low intake of selenium, a trace mineral needed for immune function, thyroid health, and cancer prevention.*[24]

❾ *Vegetarian diets are high in grains and insoluble fiber that contain phytates.* Phytates block absorption of important minerals such as calcium and zinc. Vegetarian diets are also low in zinc. Low intakes of zinc can lead to increased levels of copper, particularly in women. Elevated levels of copper in women are associated with burnout.

❿ *Strict vegetarian diets are low in vitamin B_{12}.* A lack of B_{12} can cause neurological problems and heart and artery disease.

I was a vegetarian for eleven years. I ate fish as well. When I returned to eating meat in 1997—combined with plenty of vegetables, which I continue to eat—I felt much better: more even in my energy and more focused mentally. Reintroducing lean meat or increasing its consumption has also helped many of my clients improve their health. Their total cholesterol and triglycerides go down, their HDL cholesterol goes up and their food cravings go away. Their energy is much better. Their sleep quality improves. Problems as diverse as hypoglycemia and periodontal disease are ameliorated. They feel like themselves again.

The main reason I do not like vegetarian diets? Because wild game is the most health-promoting food we have.

The Need for Optimal Health

Part of the trouble is that I've never properly understood that some disasters accumulate, that they don't all land like a child out of an apple tree.

—Janet Burroway, American writer

All degenerative disease is caused by a lack of optimal nutrition, and optimal nutrition is crucial for the attainment of optimal health.

Few people have optimal health because few pursue it. There are really two basic versions of health in our society:

➤ The "I feel all right today so I am not going to ask any questions" health. I may have disease around the corner, but if I can get through today, keep the junk food and pain relievers coming.

➤ The higher level of health: one that is not satisfied unless well-being and protection against disease are maximal.

Is there a need for optimal health? Depends on what you want out of life. If you expect to die of heart disease or cancer, or let your life end with osteoporosis or Alzheimer's disease, and are resigned to it, there is no need for optimal health. If you are convinced that nothing you can do will influence your genetic tendencies for disease, you do not need optimal health. But if you want to do everything possible to make your body resistant to disease—whatever your genetic cards may hold for you—you will want optimal health.

And that is precisely what optimal health is: optimal protection, insofar as nutrition and lifestyle will allow, against your own genetic weaknesses. That we all have genetic weaknesses is clear. But optimal nutrition, not gene therapy, is our best defense against weaknesses in our DNA. Always has been and always will be. Sorry, gene scientists.

Is it nice to know your genetic tendencies? Yes. Do we really need to? No. We should all be pursuing optimal health anyway, whether an expensive test will one day allow us to know whether or not we have an increased risk of breast cancer, heart disease, or Alzheimer's. The same strategy of optimal health will help prevent them all.

The nineteenth-century American writer Henry James called a wealthy man "one who has enough money to give him the freedom to do what he wants." This is a relative, not absolute, definition. It means that there will be different amounts for different people. And that there will also be freedom. So here are our two important nutrition points about optimal health:

➤ For cells to be optimally healthy, they need to have the freedom to have as much of all essential nutrients as possible.

➤ The amount of nutrients needed by cells to be optimally healthy will differ for each person.

Optimal health is therefore the state in which the cells of the body have enough of each nutrient to give them the freedom to do what they want. If cells want a certain amount of vitamin E to protect themselves, they should have that amount daily. If they should need so much vitamin C for immune defense or detoxification, it should be there in that amount—whether we get it through food or supplements. And, importantly, if cells need a certain balance of all nutrients, they should have that, too.

The optimal intake levels for all nutrients have not been determined. But we know they are more than the levels for merely avoiding deficiency. Just like a jet has no absolute optimal altitude, but a range in which it flies best, the optimal intake for any nutrient is going to be defined as a range. A jet can fly at one hundred feet off the ground, but for optimal speed and safety, it does better closer to thirty-five thousand feet. Merely taking enough of a nutrient to avoid deficiency is like flying at one hundred feet. You may not be grounded in deficiency, but you are not soaring with health.

Protein for growth and immune defense? Cells should have as much as they need. Fatty acids and phospholipids for all their various functions? Vitamins and minerals for a wide variety of functions? May cells have whichever they like, freely, and in whatever amount they want. This lets our genes maximize our potential for longevity and express our health to the utmost. Like the artist who needs a patron to express her talent, your cells need you to generously support them into nutritional freedom. Only then can they realize their maximal health and wellness throughout a long and healthy life.

MERELY AVOIDING DEFICIENCY IS PASSÉ

The goal of merely avoiding deficiency is passé. The real power of nutrients surfaces when we consume them in optimal amounts. A recent study of 1,312 people given selenium showed this. The study subjects were given 200 mcg per day of selenium for ten years. This resulted in a decrease in cancer deaths by 50 percent. Most important of all, this population was not selenium-deficient when the study began. This study showed clearly that the cancer-preventing power of selenium only surfaces when it is consumed in optimal— not deficiency-preventing—amounts.[25]

Such optimal nutrition allows our cells to protect themselves to the best of their ability. When our cells are free, we are free—from disease and the ravages of premature aging, which in civilized nations we mistakenly call aging. Calling heart disease, cancer, arthritis, osteoporosis, and cataracts an inevitable part of aging is like calling getting hit by a truck an inevitable part of crossing the street. They aren't if you do it right.

Cells free to do what they want are cells free from disease. Cells do not choose disease but are forced into it. Every one of us has a biochemical individuality that calls for more of a particular nutrient. That is the way our metabolism is. We will either optimize our nutrient intake to meet our needs or get a degenerative disease because these nutritional needs go unmet. The real solution to disease prevention is not to merely try to avoid disease, but to promote optimal health to the point where disease has a much harder time happening. The way we see the problem *is* the problem. We are trying to prevent individual diseases with strategies that do not work, instead of creating health on an optimal level by nourishing our body generously. As Thoreau said, "For every thousand hacking at the leaves of evil, there is one striking at the root." Promoting optimal health is the only way to strike at the root of the problem of modern degenerative diseases.

The Idea of Optimal Health

You got to be careful if you don't know where you're going, because you might not get there.

—Yogi Berra

Ideas are powerful. Without them we accomplish nothing, because without them we do not know what we want.

Take progress. This idea did not exist twelve hundred years ago in Europe in a period known as the Middle Ages. Particularly from the years 500 to 800, life was short and brutish. Merely staying alive was the main goal. Besides plague and famine, people were constantly terrorized by bands of ruthless invaders.

The idea of progress did not exist then, but in the centuries that followed, things in Europe began to change. Living conditions improved, as did the economy, and people began to realize that things could get better. They began to believe in progress because they saw it happen. Such a belief spread among all classes of people, as military service and business became two avenues through which men in particular could improve their status in society. Believing in progress and acting on their belief, Europeans eventually ushered in an age of artistic, intellectual, and economic accomplishment we call the Renaissance.

The same problem confronts us now with our health. Few know optimal health exists, so few pursue it. Because so many of us are chronically ill or marginally well, we do not even consider optimal health a possibility. The comedian Jackie Mason says that today "getting old is not so much trying to stay well but picking a disease you like." This is because we live in the dark ages of health when marauding bands of refined food companies and drug-touting physicians rule the landscape. Medicine advances but our health does not. We may be living longer, but we do so in large part by extending the lives of diseased people, not by promoting optimal wellness in the healthy.

Our goal should be to maintain optimal wellness throughout life. In the future, we will live to a hundred on average. If we employ all our faculties into truly promoting health, those will be one hundred vibrant years. We don't want to end life exhausted and riddled with our share of chronic illnesses as is the case today. We should know what it is like to enjoy life every day we are alive—and we can.

But we still continue to set our sights too low. Like the peasant from the 800s who merely wants to stay alive, we hope only to go through life and avoid serious disease, or at least to slow down its progression with drugs. We don't know that we should seek abundant health because we have never had it, just as the peasant does not miss the pleasures and safety of modern times because he has never had them.

We must first realize that abundant health can be had and enjoyed throughout life, and that to have it we must make it happen. In dreams begin responsibilities. To bring our vision of optimal health into fruition, we must optimize the health of our body throughout life with the tools available to us. The responsibilities of optimal health require that we eat a diet of whole foods, take supplements, exercise, manage stress, and seek spiritual wellness. We must spend money preventively if we wish to not spend it on heroic treatments that are too little and too late. We must see such a diversion of resources to aggressive preventive medicine as the most logical approach to disease prevention. We must do this as individuals even in the face of a culture that does not take such long-term goals like optimal health seriously. We must do this even though our media and scientific culture is filled with short-sighted researchers who do not realize that there is already enough evidence to suggest we ought to do so.

We will not be the suppressed sick of the world, whose illnesses are covered by medications. We will be the truly healthy, whose vibrancy comes from giving the cells of our body what they want—nutrients—and not what they struggle to avoid—drugs. The diseases we die from are not drug deficiencies. To treat them as such is to guarantee of failure. All chronic diseases are caused by the drugs purported to treat them or a lack of an optimal supply of nutrients, exercise, or spiritual wellness.

We first have to believe that optimal health exists and is worth pursuing. Then the idea of optimal health will take root in our society. When it does, optimal health will be as second nature to us as the idea of progress is now.

Energizing vs. Protective Nutrients

The era of nutrient supplements to promote health and reduce illness is here to stay.

—Ranjit Chandra, M.D., *Journal of the American Medical Association*, May 7, 1997

Everybody loves antioxidants. That's because antioxidants are protective nutrients that promote the healthy use of oxygen by the body. They help prevent many diseases, most notably heart disease. They appear to slow the aging process. They include nutrients such as vitamins C and E, selenium, zinc, and N-acetyl-cysteine. But as wonderful as antioxidants are, they don't do everything.

Let's return to our medieval town. To stay alive it must be able to protect itself from invaders. To do that you would want to build a strong city wall, but a wall alone will not keep a city vibrant. You must also stimulate the life of that city and its economy. Only then will the city thrive.

So it is with our cells. We live in an age when marauding cellular invaders dominate our environment. Smog, cigarette smoke, stress, refined vegetable oils, margarine, and fried foods are all treacherous to the health of the cellular community. The nutrition field has been right to want to armor our cells with the right protective nutrients. Yet we need to be equally concerned about increasing cellular energy, the lifeblood of our cells.

Protection and energy are interrelated. A cell with more energy is better able to protect itself and build a stronger wall against invaders. Good antioxidant nutrients protect the energy-manufacturing ability of our cells, so the two strategies work hand in hand.

We must not forget the energizing part of our health strategy. A well-protected cell without vitality will die too soon, though it be well-armed. Defense alone cannot keep our cells healthy. They also must have a good offense: energy.

Energizing our cells may be even more important than protecting them. This is partly due to the fact that energizing our cells makes them better able to protect themselves. Without energy, cells cannot live. If you run out of energy, you take a nap. If a cell runs out of energy, it dies. We can't let that happen, especially in key areas of the body where new cells are in short supply, such as in the brain and the heart.

These are the cell-energizing nutrients that we need to pay more attention to:

The Cell-Energizing Superstars
➤ *Carnitine*
➤ *Acetyl-L-Carnitine*
➤ *CoQ10*
➤ *The B complex vitamins*
➤ *Magnesium*
➤ *Lipoic acid*
➤ *Flaxseed oil*
➤ *The fatty acids EPA and DHA*
➤ *Medium chain triglycerides (MCTs)*

MITOCHONDRIA: BODY ENERGIZERS

Mitochondria are like cells within your cells. They are small, rodlike structures that handle much of the process of turning food into energy. They are present in all the cells of the body except mature red blood cells.

Mitochondria are powerhouses. They are nonstop parties, nightclubs that never close, supplying 90 percent of the energy that is driving your cells. The more active your body, the more mitochondria you have. The healthier you are, the more energy they make. When they start to fade, you do, too.

Why are they so important? Nearly all of the energy in your body comes from them. Without them, you cannot live. If they are tired, you are, too. If you energize them naturally with carnitine and CoQ10, however, you will have a lot more energy.

(continued on next page)

(continued from previous page)

As we age, our mitochondria make less energy. Like parties that have gone on too long, they become slower and more boring. Boring, less-energetic mitochondria make for cells more prone to disease. Cells with more fatigued mitochondria age more quickly. Liven up your mitochondria with the right nutrients, however, and you will slow the aging process. In other words, the more energized your cells, the longer your life and the more freedom from disease you will have.

The most important nutrient for increasing mitochondrial energy and efficiency is carnitine. Carnitine keeps energizing compounds coming into the mitochondrial party. It also acts like a bouncer and quickly gets rid of anything that could slow the party down.

A fish rots from the head down. The cells of your body rot from the mitochondria out. You are only as young and energetic as your mitochondria.[26] To appreciate the importance of the mitochondria in your body, think of your heart. It keeps your body fed with oxygen and food and speeds away waste products. The same could be said of the mitochondria. They feed the cells they inhabit. If we keep mitochondria happy, we will be happy. The way to do that is with nutrients like carnitine.

How young are you? As young as your mitochondria.

We need both protective and energizing nutrients for optimal health. And how we get our energy is important. We can get it naturally through enhancing the natural way our cells work, or we can stimulate our cells artificially, which I do not recommend.

While supplements are crucial, there are more basic things we need to do first to maximize energy. Let's look at them.

Top Ten Ways to Maximize Energy Naturally

❶ *Eat enough protein.* This is one of the most important ways to keep blood sugar balanced and energy levels high. Two to three meals per day that contain protein is best for most people. Make sure to eat some protein with breakfast to get your body off to the right start.

❷ *Limit sugar intake as much as possible.* Sugar may give you instant energy, but in the long term it will only make you more tired.

❸ *Don't work too much.* Easier said than done. This is one of the main causes of fatigue. Everyone should take vacations and have plenty of leisure activity—not alternate work activity—on the weekends.

❹ *Get enough sleep.* This means being able to wake up without an alarm clock to get you going.

❺ *Don't exercise too much, too little, or too intensely.* All three will make you tired. If you are a stressed-out person, don't pick a stressful form of exercise such as running or aerobics. Try Tai Chi, yoga, hiking, or walking. The general rule with exercise is that it should leave you refreshed, not wiped out. Walking is the best way to start.

❻ *Check for food allergies.* Eating foods your body is allergic or sensitive to—wheat and dairy are common offenders—can cause fatigue. If there is a food you love and eat every day, eliminate it for two weeks and see if your energy increases.

❼ *Make sure you do not have a yeast overgrowth or other digestive disturbance.* Gas, bloating, spaciness, and carbohydrate cravings often accompany such problems. A nutritionist or nutritionally oriented practitioner can help you determine whether this may be the case.

❽ *Make sure you do not have any medical conditions that can cause fatigue.* These include low thyroid function, hemochromatosis (iron-storage disease), and a range of other ailments.

❾ *Resolve emotional and spiritual issues.* This is important for avoiding the stress and worry that can reduce sleep quality and excessively stress the body.

❿ *Take supplements.* Food does not give us enough carnitine, CoQ10, magnesium, and other key energizing nutrients we need for optimal energy levels. Let's look at these in depth.

Energizing Nutrients

Carnitine is without a doubt the most important nutrient for increasing energy levels naturally. But let's look at some of the other energizing nutrients and see how they work along with carnitine. The key here is that these are nutrients and not stimulants— they are natural to the body and will have only beneficial effects over the short and long term.

Don't think you need to take all of these nutrients for maximal energy. Start with carnitine, antioxidants, and flaxseed oil, and build from there as your energy requirements dictate.

Carnitine

The most powerful energizing nutrient. Doses of 500 to 4,000 mg per day of pure carnitine from carnitine tartrate can be used. Start with 500 mg per day and increase dosage by 500 mg per day until you achieve your desired energy level.

CoQ10

CoQ10 naturally energizes the body, increases heart health, enhances immune function, and promotes weight loss. CoQ10 is a close partner to carnitine in the body, and it almost always follows that where carnitine will be beneficial, CoQ10 will be as well.

For promoting energy, most people take 30 to 100 mg per day. For more severe fatigue, doses of 100 to 300 mg are recommended. Doses of 400 mg of CoQ10 have been found to reverse breast cancer according to published case histories.[27]

Flaxseed Oil

Both freshly ground flaxseeds and flaxseed oil are very energizing. One tablespoon of flaxseed oil or three tablespoons of freshly ground flaxmeal per day is the amount I most often recommend. It is so energizing that if you consume it too close to bedtime, you may have difficulty falling asleep!

B Complex

This family of vitamins is well known for its ability to help the body turn food into energy. Many people find that 50 to 100 mg of B complex helps maximize energy. I have seen clinically that it often takes at least 50 mg of B complex vitamins to have a noticeable effect on energy levels, particularly in people over forty. A 50 mg B vitamin complex will typically have 50 mg of B_1, B_2, niacinamide, pantothenic acid, and B_6, with 400 mcg of folic acid and 50 mcg of B_{12}. A high-dose multivitamin may also offer these amounts.

Magnesium

Every time your body wants to make energy, you need magnesium. A lack of magnesium is a common cause of fatigue. Most forms of magnesium are effective, and I usually recommend 400 to 600 mg per day. For the most energizing effects of magnesium, you may want to try magnesium malate. This is because the malic acid that gives it the name "malate" is also energizing.

Malic Acid

If the body does not have enough oxygen in it, it has trouble breaking down food and using it for energy. One of the nutrients that can help buffer this effect of low oxygen is malic acid. This is because malic acid can work both in the presence and absence of oxygen to help the body get the most energy from food.

Malic acid in doses of 1,200 to 2,400 mg has been found to relieve muscle pain associated with fibromyalgia, perhaps by increasing energy metabolism and decreasing muscle breakdown. Animal studies have shown that malic acid increases energy levels and endurance. Malic acid deserves more study and holds great promise as a natural energizer.

Medium Chain Triglycerides (MCTs)

MCTs, which stands for medium chain triglycerides, are fats with unique properties. MCTs are very easily burned by the body and are very helpful for those who want extra energy, especially during competitive sports. They can also be used to help promote energy in those who are in ketosis. The liquid form is the most economical, although MCTs are available in capsules as well. I usually recommend one teaspoon to one tablespoon per day with breakfast. One of the nice side effects of the increased energy people experience with MCTs is that it greatly increases their urge to exercise. MCTs can be used for cooking, although I do not recommend you fry with MCTs.

Antioxidants: Vitamins C and E

Vitamins C and E play an important role in helping maintain red blood cell health which is crucial for oxygen transfer in the body and maximum energy levels. These antioxidants also protect against the build up of free radicals in the body. Free radicals in excess are often one of the main causes of fatigue. Minimum doses for everyone should be 1,000 mg of vitamin C and 400 IUs of vitamin E. I have often seen people who are so loaded with free radicals that they have greatly increased energy after just adding these two supplements to their diet.

Lipoic Acid

Lipoic acid helps the body use fats and carbohydrates better for energy. It also protects the energy cycles of cells from coming "unhooked," and therefore keeps cells maximally energized. Lipoic acid is also a powerful antioxidant. Doses of 50 to 200 mg help maximize energy.

NADH

NADH is a very special form of the B vitamin niacinamide and has only recently become available. Most people do not need to take NADH, which is at present a very expensive supplement. But for those with severe fatigue, Parkinson's disease, or any other chronic health problem, NADH can be helpful and sometimes remarkably energizing. NADH also helps enhance short-term memory and alleviates depression. Usual doses are between 2.5 and 10 mg per day for those who can afford this remarkable nutrient.

Natural Energy vs. Stimulant Energy

You can increase your energy in two ways. One builds the body up. The other destroys it.

Energizing nutrients and herbs work by naturally supporting the energy-releasing highways of the body. They naturally optimize the mitochondria's ability to turn food into energy. These natural compounds do not stress the body, but maximize its natural energy pathways. Using them is a win-win situation.

Stimulants, on the other hand, weaken you. They push the body too far—usually farther than the body wants to go. They stimulate central nervous system function, and in so doing are not really nutritional or "natural" in any sense. Used regularly, they wear the body down. When abused, they are destructive.

Natural Energizing Nutrients	Drug-like Stimulants
Carnitine	Coffee (caffeinated)
CoQ10	Kola nut
Flaxseed oil	Guarana
B complex	Ephedra (also known as Ma Huang)
Magnesium	
Malic acid	
MCTs	
Antioxidants	
Lipoic acid	
NADH	

Energy is best increased in the body by naturally supporting the body's energy pathways, not by whipping the glands and central nervous system with stimulants. Let's look at the difference in effects of these two kinds of energizing substances sold in health food stores:

	Stimulants Examples: ephedra and kola nut standardized extracts	Energizing Nutrients Examples: carnitine, CoQ10, lipoic acid
Method of Energy Increase	Stimulate central nervous system	Natural: promote optimal function of energy pathways in the body
Addictive	Yes	No
Quality of Energy	Jittery, stimulant energy	Natural, even energy
Short-Term Effects	Initial energy burst, then fatigue	Natural increase in energy that only improves over time
Long-Term Effects	Burns out adrenal glands; long-term use lowers energy and possibly immunity; may accelerate aging process	Increase energy with no adverse effects. Increase immune function; may slow aging process
Other uses	Ephedra can offer acute relief from asthma attack	Optimize many aspects of mitochondrial function; promote heart health; quench free radicals; maximize cellular health
Side Effects	Worsen hypertension and diabetes; promote and/or aggravate arrhythmias	None
Normal Constituents of Human Metabolism?	No	Yes

Ephedra

Ephedra has long been used for the relief of asthma. This is a responsible and appropriate use of this herb. Often, the plant is used in an alcohol-based tincture and is balanced with herbs such as licorice to help even out its effects on the body.

What is unfortunately being touted by many companies, however, is a standardized extract of ephedra, which is as different from an alcohol tincture as a missile is from a slingshot. Standardizing the plant for its most powerful constituents is taking the herb out of context and creating a brutish supplement that pushes the body into overdrive. I have seen many examples where the short- and long-term use of these ephedra extracts have caused harm.

I had a client who was very fond of the power of standardized ephedra products to help her lose weight. Against my advice, she used them and lost weight more quickly. Yet after six months, the product did not help her any more. Then she began gaining weight she could not lose. I have seen this time and again, and warn people that the long-term use of these ephedra extracts can quickly put you into a metabolic prison from which it is difficult if not impossible to escape. Taking these powerful ephedra extracts is like crying wolf on a daily basis to your sympathetic nervous system, the "fight or flight" part of the autonomic or unconscious nervous system. This part of the body has a strong influence over how the body loses weight. Stimulate this part of the nervous system too much and too often and you may find that it no longer has the strength to do the job it once did. Suddenly, weight loss and energy are further from you than ever before.

Adrenal exhaustion—also known as burnout—is an epidemic in this country. These ephedra products stress our adrenal glands even more and only make this problem worse.

And why use ephedra to lose weight when we have carnitine, which works much better and is completely beneficial?

Carnitine Enhances Sports Performance

Fat is the best fuel for endurance exercise. While you can burn off all the stored carbohydrates during the course of a single marathon, you have enough fat on your body to run for days. While carbohydrates play an important role in promoting endurance, fat is the most abundant source of energy in the body. Therefore, optimizing the body's ability to burn fat is the most important thing an endurance athlete can do to promote energy and endurance.

Carnitine, which plays such a critical role in fat-burning, might seem like something that would greatly enhance performance in endurance athletics. Sometimes it does, and sometimes it doesn't. Why? It depends on the many different variables in the way carnitine is used.

➤ *People who are most out of shape will benefit remarkably from carnitine supplements. Highly trained athletes will benefit as well, though they may not notice the same dramatic increase in performance out-of-shape exercisers will.*

➤ *If endurance and performance are not enhanced by carnitine, there may be problems with the purity of the product used. Pure L-carnitine tartrate works best, while other forms that are not as pure do not always work as well. This conclusion comes from my experience working with athletes. Switching to the tartrate form can greatly increase the results in performance enhancement.*

➤ *People often do not take enough carnitine to get its full benefits. I see some people who benefit from 500 to 1,000 mg per day, while others need 4 grams per day to see an effect on maximal performance and endurance. Little or no effect will be seen with a dose of 250 mg of carnitine.*

Much research points to the benefits of carnitine in endurance sports. Carnitine enhances aerobic performance, allowing athletes to exercise longer without fatigue.[28] Another study showed that a group of trained runners given 2 grams of carnitine per day increased their peak running speed by a remarkable 5.7 percent.[29]

One of the most frequent comments I hear from my clients is that they have much better athletic endurance when they take carnitine regularly. This is particularly true for those who only exercise once or twice per week. Research corroborates this, showing that carnitine can stimulate the efficient use of fat as fuel in nontrained athletes to give them that "trained-like" state of greater endurance.[30]

Carnitine also helps elite performers. A study of 110 trained athletes showed that carnitine helps improve endurance.[31] The dose that appears to be most helpful is in the range of 1 to 4 grams per day. Carnitine is most effective when taken for a few weeks prior to competition. Some studies even show that carnitine increases muscle strength in endurance athletes. This may be because carnitine helps burn fat for energy, thus sparing the muscle tissue that is sometimes broken down and used for fuel during intense aerobic sports.[32]

CARNITINE CASE HISTORY

I put Tara, thirty-four, on 2,000 mg of carnitine per day. She saw a slight increase in weight loss, but what she loved the most was the abundant energy she now felt. When she went to work out at the gym, she now had so much stamina that she stayed on the treadmill for a full hour. She had previously become fatigued after thirty minutes of jogging. She also loved the fact that she no longer felt the 4:00 P.M. energy crunch that once sent her to the candy machine or the pastry shop. Carnitine also gave her the energy to exercise every day, which she loved to do.

Carnitine is also recommended for athletes because running and intense aerobics increase carnitine loss in the urine.[33] Many kinds of training decrease body carnitine levels, and carnitine supplements make up for this loss.[34]

Another important advantage of carnitine is that it prevents muscle damage during vigorous exercise, especially in those who are not trained athletes. Three grams of carnitine per day taken for three to six weeks significantly reduced muscle pain and tenderness after exercise in a group of six untrained adults. Signs of protein breakdown in muscle were also reduced.[35] Carnitine also decreases the formation of damaged fats known as lipid peroxides during exercise, further evidence that it protects cells during sports.[36]

One of the most useful things carnitine does to promote endurance is to maximize the speed of lactate use by the body. When the body makes a lot of lactate during intense sports like running and cycling, you can feel a "burn" in your legs that slows you down. Carnitine helps promote the metabolism of lactate into energy, and helps delay the onset of the lactate burn. This is important not only for preventing the accumulation of this irritant that slows down performance, but because it also turns lactate into something that the body can use for energy.[37] Many studies have confirmed that carnitine both increases aerobic output and decreases lactate accumulation.[38] This promotion of lactate use may be the most important thing carnitine does to enhance sports performance.[39] Indeed, in top athletes, carnitine increases overall performance through avenues other than enhanced fat-burning, and this increased use of lactate is one of them.[40] The many ways in which carnitine energizes the body are still being discovered.

Another area where carnitine is also useful—although we do not know why—is in carbohydrate metabolism. Carnitine is found in large quantities in the flight muscles of flies. These muscles use carbohydrates rather than fatty acids. Acetyl-L-carnitine in particular appears to be important in maximizing carbohydrate metabolism.[41] Athletes may therefore want to take both L-carnitine and acetyl-L-carnitine to get all the benefits carnitine offers for maximizing sports performance. Taking both will optimize both the fat- and carbohydrate-burning metabolic pathways and optimally energize the body.

Older adults benefit greatly from carnitine during exercise. Carnitine levels decline with age, and because of this, fatty acids can accumulate, making the energy pathways of the cell sluggish.[42] For these and many other reasons, carnitine is a must supplement for those over forty who want to maximize their energy and exercise endurance.

For those undergoing hemodialysis, or for those with intermittent claudication, carnitine can help make exercise such as walking possible. Those with heart conditions such as angina and cardiomyopathy should also supplement with carnitine and CoQ10 to help them do whatever exercise their doctor recommends.[43]

WHEN TO TAKE CARNITINE

You should take carnitine daily to keep muscles primed, and extra carnitine before an endurance event to keep the body optimally able to release energy. The peak of carnitine in your blood plasma occurs thirty to sixty minutes after you take it. Blood levels are really not as important, however, as the amount of carnitine inside your muscles and the amount in the carnitine-dependent enzymes in your cells. This can take weeks to build up.

To help enhance athletic performance, start with one gram (1,000 mg) of carnitine per day in divided doses before breakfast and lunch. Increase your dose, if needed, by an additional one gram every week until you see a difference in endurance and performance. Most athletes find that between one and four grams is helpful. Do not take carnitine too late in the day or it may keep you awake at night! I usually recommend that people do not take carnitine much later than lunchtime to avoid too much late-night energy.

Carnitine plays countless roles helping the body turn food into energy, all of them natural and beneficial. For sports where any level of endurance is involved, and especially for the occasional runner, tennis player, or basketball player, carnitine can enhance your endurance. If you are an older adult, your tissues have less carnitine and you will benefit even more. If you are an elite athlete, you may just shave a few seconds off your time that could make all the difference in the world.

TOP TEN WAYS CARNITINE ENHANCES SPORTS PERFORMANCE

To sum up then, here are the most important reasons why carnitine should be taken by both occasional and professional athletes. Sorry for the technical language, but sports folks like to know the details:

❶ *Carnitine helps the body become more metabolically efficient in a large number of ways,* all of which benefit athletic performance.

❷ *Carnitine helps the body burn more fat during endurance exercise.*

❸ *Carnitine enhances carbohydrate metabolism,* helping the body burn sugars more effectively as well.

❹ *Carnitine lowers the lactate-to-pyruvate ratio.* This enhances metabolic efficiency and therefore energy production in muscle cells. More pyruvate will be available for energy production, and less lactate will build up to cause the "burn" that slows performance.

❺ *Optimal levels of carnitine lower levels of acetyl CoA in the mitochondria that build up during exercise.* Excess acetyl CoA gums up the mitochondria and slows energy production.

❻ *Carnitine directly increases the activity of respiratory chain (energy-releasing) enzymes in muscles,* therefore increasing the ability of the body to make energy.

❼ *Carnitine reduces muscle pain and tenderness after exercise.*

❽ *Carnitine reduces heart rate during exercise,* especially at maximum workload.

❾ *Carnitine helps untrained athletes exercise longer,* especially those who have limited endurance.

❿ *Carnitine prevents the formation of lipid peroxides during exercise,* protecting tissues from free radicals during endurance sports.

Carnitine: The Best Nutrient for Weight Loss

For most of the population, the concentration of carnitine is the most important factor governing the rate of fat metabolism.

— Brian Leibovitz, Ph.D.

Garage sales are great. They help you turn what you don't need any more into ready cash. And often the money that comes from these garage sales goes into refurbishing the house. Carnitine puts on a nutritional garage sale. It rids the body of excess fat and other fatty acid residues that are only getting in the way. And it creates the cellular equivalent of cash: energy. This energy often goes into repairing and refurbishing the cells of our body.

Turning fat into energy is the greatest conversion that can be made in the body. And only carnitine can make it happen.

Imagine that you have an idiosyncratic overweight neighbor named Phil. Phil's car isn't well maintained. When it comes down the street, the exhaust creates a cloud. Phil keeps putting gas in the tank. He even loads extra cans of gas into the trunk just to be sure he never runs out. The car is so loaded up with gas that you hope it doesn't explode. What you can't understand is why Phil doesn't stop putting fuel in the car and give it what it needs: a tune-up!

This car has more potential energy than any car you know. You cannot figure out why in the world he would spend all that time loading it with gas, and yet not give it new spark plugs. The funny thing is, Phil drives the car around figuring that if he puts enough gas in it and keeps driving it around, the car's problems will work themselves out.

Phil's car is just like his overweight body: too much energy and not enough nutrients (spark plugs) to burn it. Seems hard to believe—paradoxical as well—that an overweight body would lack nutrients. But we are not talking about the big nutrients like fat, protein, and carbohydrates. We are talking about the nutrients that don't have calories and that are needed in smaller amounts: vitamins, minerals, and nutrients like carnitine.

Nutrients won't do everything. You need a diet that allows for a lower insulin level, and that simply means a diet lower in carbohydrates and higher in protein. Exercise is also important. But exercise alone will not solve Phil's nutrient-related problems any more than driving a car around will tune it up.

Tuning up your metabolism with the right nutrients is essential for weight loss. There is significant scientific evidence that increased levels of carnitine in tissues leads to increased fat burning.[44] Carnitine is the forklift that takes fat to the fat incinerators in our cells called mitochondria. Unless fat makes it into the mitochondria, you can't burn it off no matter what you do and no matter how well you diet. Once fat is inside the mitochondria, fat is magically transformed into energy. It's like turning bricks into gold. This is why carnitine both encourages weight loss and increases energy levels.[45]

Carnitine also helps increase metabolic rate while also maintaining the amount of muscle tissue—important advantages for long-term weight loss.[46] Carnitine is also one of the most important nutrients for keeping blood sugar constant and eliminating cravings.[47]

Carnitine is particularly helpful for anyone on a low carbohydrate diet. Without carnitine, low carbohydrate diets can lead to fatigue and food cravings. Yet with 500 to 2,000 mg of carnitine per day, these diets become much easier to stay on, for energy levels increase and cravings lessen.

CARNITINE INCREASES WEIGHT LOSS ELEVENFOLD

A recent study of overweight teenagers showed the powerful advantage of using carnitine. For those eating a healthy diet and getting moderate exercise for twelve weeks, the average weight loss was one pound. For those who added one gram of carnitine per day to the same regime, weight loss averaged eleven pounds! This is the most dramatic study to date showing the power of a single nutrient to promote weight loss.[48]

Top Ten Things to Do to Lose Weight Permanently

❶ *Eat protein at each meal.* This is the single most important thing. I am going to say this many times in this book, because inadequate protein intake is the single most important mistake made by people who are overweight, women in particular. It is this misguided fear of protein and love of carbohydrates that causes most of the obesity in this country.

❷ *Eat protein at each meal.* See, I said it again. I wasn't kidding. I only have ten things on this list, and I have used up two of them already. So please get enough protein, which means having it in regular amounts at each meal. You have a lot of ways to get protein: fish, goat cheese, almonds, turkey, flank steak, chicken breast: whatever you like, and spread it out throughout the day. Let your appetite tell you when you have eaten enough. Four ounces—a serving the size of a deck of cards—two to three times per day works best for most people. You may need more.

❸ *Eat quality fats.* People crave fats because they are missing the omega-3 fats their body needs. These are found in salmon, sardines, mackerel, albacore tuna, nuts and seeds of all kinds as well as flaxseed, canola, and walnut oil. If you do not like any of these foods, softgel omega-3 fatty acid supplements are available.

❹ *Don't eat a "fat-free" diet.* There is no culture in the world that has ever eaten a fat-free diet. The fattest people I know are those who eat nothing but high-sugar, fat-free foods. Fats are essential for health and weight loss. A diet that tries to be fat-free is invariably one with too many carbohydrates. Excessive starches and sugars in the diet turn into fat in the body, thus making fat-free diets Trojan horse "fat-laden" diets. These diets are really the best way to gain weight and create ill health. Cattle, after all, are fattened by being fed a low-fat diet high in carbohydrates—grains.

❺ *Don't weigh or otherwise try to accurately measure your food intake—just use common sense, limit your carbohydrates, and use Paleolithic principles.* If you eat enough protein and healthy fats, and keep sugar and grain products to a minimum, you will be eating what humans have eaten for millennia. Your body will respond happily by saying, "Hey, I know what this stuff is. I've had enough!" High carbohydrate foods such as grains, bread, pasta, sugar, and candy, however, are new to the body, so it takes much longer for it to know when to stop asking for food. You can be on your third plate of pasta, and your 100,000-year-old digestive tract will still be trying to figure out what it is, let alone tell you that it is satisfied with what you have eaten.

❻ *Take carnitine.* The key is to take enough, and get the right quality carnitine, carnitine tartrate. Take 500 to 2,000 mg of carnitine per day, usually before breakfast and lunch for the best results.

❼ *Exercise.* I read women's magazines constantly. I do this to see what kind of nutrition information they have. I never look at the photos of beautiful women. Really. In every issue I see pictures of women exercising. I have asked many women who read these magazines if they have ever done these exercises. They say no. No one ever has. The problem with these photos is that looking at them makes women feel as though they have exercised. So I say, no more photos of women exercising. At least in women's magazines.

Don't defeat yourself. Don't look at things that make you feel like you exercised. (Guys do this every Sunday watching football.) Actually do a few minutes of exercise per day—in a way that you enjoy and find fun.

Exercise fun? It used to be. Before the modern day puritans invented aerobics and told us to "go for the burn" and "no pain, no gain," people burned fat without a burning sensation and had lots of gain with little pain. There are a million ways to get fit, all of them fun. And people once moved their bodies only because they enjoyed the experience. Dancing, hiking, skiing— the fact that it was good for you was never mentioned.

Exercise only because you enjoy it. Don't motivate yourself by aping surgically altered former actresses who are selling you videos under the false pretense that their eternal physique comes from their special exercises. This kind of motivation ends after you get tired of looking at the picture on the box. Bowling, dancing, bowling and dancing at the same time—do what you like. Hiking. Walking around your neighborhood and meeting the people who live near you. Well, maybe hiking.

Pick something you like to do that's fun that involves body movement. Don't think of it as exercise or you won't do it. Don't set a specified amount of time that you make yourself exercise. This works for dedicated athletes but is a killjoy for the rest of us. Move your body as long as it remains fun and stop the minute it isn't. Let fun be your guide and fun you'll have.

Anything is better than nothing. The greatest darkness must yield to the smallest light, and anything you can do—walking to the corner for the paper instead of driving—is a great start.

8 *Don't be in a hurry to lose weight.* Life is long. You have lots of time to lose weight. The more slowly you do it, the more permanently you will keep it off. People are much more impressed with how permanently we lose weight than how quickly.

The less stress you put yourself under during weight loss the better. Quick weight loss is stressful physically, emotionally, and mentally. Stress ages you, and actually makes weight loss more difficult. Slower weight loss—about a pound or two a week—is often more permanent. Take your time.

9 *Enjoy your meals.* If you don't, you will develop a pleasure deficiency. Pleasure is the most important nutrient of all, for it feeds the soul. A pleasure deficiency will push you off your diet faster than anything else.

10 *Eat a diet that is suited to your unique needs.* Ancestry, activity levels, stress levels, present nutrient levels in your body and your biochemical individuality—all of these dictate what you need in the way of food and supplements. Ideally, this would be designed for you by a nutritionist who could perform various metabolic tests. Not everyone can afford this, but for those who can it is well worth the investment. The many menu plans in this book may be helpful, but there is nothing better than something tailored to your needs. If you can't see a nutritionist, become your own: experiment and make note of which foods and combinations of foods make you feel best. Listen to your body, and it will guide you aright.

The Value of a Low Carbohydrate Diet

If I had to choose one single therapeutic tool to reduce the suffering of chronically ill patients, no matter what the nature or cause of their illness, I would opt for a reduction of excessive intake of simple carbohydrates, not only those found in "junk" foods such as candies and pastries, but also those found in "healthy" foods such as whole grain-breads and fruits. Of course, not all chronically ill patients ingest inappropriately high amounts of simple carbohydrates. However, when they do, which, in this country, is generally the rule, my experience suggests that chronic symptomatology of virtually any type will improve dramatically within 30 to 60 days when intake is significantly reduced.

> —Dr. Jeffrey Moss, Certified Nutrition Specialist

The general imprecise way of observing sees everywhere in nature opposites (for example, warm and cold) where there are not opposites, but differences of degree. An unspeakable amount of painfulness, arrogance, harshness, estrangement, and frigidity has entered into human feelings because we think we see opposites instead of transitions.

> —Friedrich Nietzsche

We need to understand that moderately decreasing our carbohydrate intake can do a lot of good. Weight loss, more energy, and lower blood cholesterol and triglyceride levels can all happen.

Carbohydrates can be beneficial. Good carbohydrates—fruits and vegetables—often are, though there are many, myself included, who feel best limiting fruit. Modern carbohydrates—grains, breads, and especially sugars—can cause problems. Most of the people who walk into my office are eating more carbohydrates than are good for them.

The problem with carbohydrates usually occurs only when we overdo it. We can consume a moderate amount and feel fine. But when my clients start to get more than half their calories from carbohydrates—grains, bread, cereal, fruits, fruit juice, candy, whatever source they choose—they get into trouble. Food cravings appear or get worse, and energy levels go down. Weight increases. Blood cholesterol and triglyceride levels worsen.

We need to transition to a more balanced intake of protein, fats, and carbohydrates. For most of my clients, their maintenance diet is around 45 percent carbohydrates, 35 percent fat, and 20 percent protein. During weight loss, when 1,200 calories are consumed daily, their diet is around 35 percent carbohydrates, 35 percent fat and 30 percent protein. These numbers do not need to be exact, and I do not recommend you try to be perfect about anything in your diet, be it these ratios or anything else. But you should start to transition in this direction. The carnitine program diet plans will get you there.

Diets with differing carbohydrate levels have remarkably different effects. This is true especially for blood cholesterol and triglyceride readings. The April 1997 *American Journal of Clinical Nutrition* featured a study comparing two groups consuming diets containing either 40 or 60 percent carbohydrates. Those with the higher carbohydrate intake had higher blood cholesterol and triglyceride readings after being on such a diet for only three weeks. The authors concluded that "there is now substantial evidence that low-fat, high-carbohydrate diets lead to changes in glucose, insulin, and lipoprotein metabolism that will increase the risk of ischemic heart disease."[49]

But if 15 percent of the carbohydrates in a high-carbohydrate diet are replaced with protein, things improve markedly. LDL goes down, HDL goes up, and triglycerides plummet. All this by lowering carbohydrate intake from 65 to 50 percent, while leaving fat at a constant of 25 percent. The difference is made up by increasing protein from 10 to 25 percent of the diet.[50]

I have implemented every diet imaginable over the past eleven years in my busy nutrition practice. For years I tried to make high-carbohydrate diets work and couldn't. In my long experience with the many types of diets available, I have opted for a more balanced diet. Most of my clients who try a high-carbohydrate diet have increased food cravings, lowered energy, worsened yeast overgrowths, food allergies, blood sugar imbalances, PMS, adrenal exhaustion, and mood disorders. In those with HIV and chronic fatigue (a large part of my practice), the effects of a high-carbohydrate diet (60 percent carbohydrates or more) have varied from the mildly negative to the disastrous. The reason I do not like high-carbohydrate diets is that in the vast majority of cases, I have found them not to work.

My present job also includes evaluating the clinical successes of over fifty nutritionists in the mid-Atlantic states area. Much of the clinical success of these nutritionists comes from decreasing carbohydrate intake, increasing quality protein while also increasing the quality of fat their clients eat. The improvements in triglycerides and HDL cholesterol have been most favorable when the diet contains no more than 40 percent carbohydrates.

I often hear many mention the work of Dean Ornish, M.D., and his assertion that a very low-fat diet high in carbohydrates can reverse heart disease. His published research, however, assesses this diet in a combination with overall lifestyle changes, including:

➤ *Stopping smoking*
➤ *Stress management*
➤ *Group support*
➤ *Moderate aerobic exercise*

His diet, therefore, was one of five things used to treat heart disease in this study. This research therefore cannot be used to support the assertion that a low-fat diet alone can reverse heart disease any more than it can be used to prove group support alone will reverse heart disease. Also, his participants received B_{12} supplements, which may have lowered homocysteine, a cholesterol-independent heart disease–causing compound in the body. Triglyceride levels went up in people in his study, which suggests there may be long-term insulin metabolism problems in those who continue on such a high-carbohydrate regime.[51]

The unanswered question about high-carbohydrate diets is: Why promote something never seen in Paleolithic nutrition? The diet that humans ate from 2.6 million years to 10,000 years ago has had on average 41 percent carbohydrates,[52] some say even less. If we have become acclimated to this level of carbohydrates in our diet over the vast majority of our history and have only become agrarian in the past five to ten thousand years, how can we hope to quickly adapt to so drastic a shift in our macronutrient intake?

The bottom line is clinical. A more balanced diet program works. More energy, better weight loss, and greater resistance to disease.

HOW MANY CARBOHYDRATES SHOULD YOU EAT?

But how do you know what amount of carbohydrates is best for you?

Experiment. Start with the carnitine program menu plans, which adhere to Paleolithic principles. Then adjust the carbohydrate intake to create something that works best for you.

If you are eating a diet high in carbohydrates, you may feel okay, but this does not mean it is the best diet for you. This is confusing to many people. They feel they are doing well on their vegetarian or high-carbohydrate regime, except that they are feeling tired, have food cravings and can't lose weight. They think this is normal because their friends who are also eating high carbohydrate diets also have these problems. This is not normal! We are designed to be healthy, vital, and trim. A program based on the Paleolithic diet will get you there.

Let's look at different people and the differing amounts of carbohydrates they do well on.

Mary is someone who feels best eating two starch servings and one fruit per day. She has a half cup of oatmeal with her eggs for breakfast, a salad of grilled chicken and spinach with dressing for lunch, and a sweet potato with her meat or fish for dinner. Mary notices that more than one fruit per day makes her feel sluggish. She feels great on just that amount of carbohydrates. If she starts eating a lot of bread or pasta, she feels tired. She knows she needs more protein and less carbohydrates to keep up with her busy job and family, and has learned that her PMS is much improved when she has more protein and less starches in her diet. She has seen the best weight loss in her life on this lower-carbohydrate regime.

Noreen feels best when she eats no bread or grain products of any kind. She feels great, is slim and energetic, and has great physical and mental energy when she eats no bread, pasta, cereal, rolls, or any other grain-based foods. Fruits do not seem to bother her, in amounts of two to three per day. Her carbohydrate sensitivity seems to occur only with grains. Avoiding them has made her feel wonderful and has solved her digestive problems of gas and bloating. She finds that nuts are a terrific snack for her. She has no problem resisting things like cakes and cookies because she is now more interested in the gourmet aspect of her meal, and she remembers how lousy she felt on the high-grain diet she once followed so avidly.

Laura is different. She has found that eating no carbohydrates— no grains, bread, pasta, or fruit—makes her feel best. It took her two years of trial and error to figure this out. But she finally has the energy she needs, looks as slim as she wants, and does not have the mood swings and depression she once had. Only after going on and off this diet many times did she realize that it was the one she should be on. Her cholesterol and triglycerides also came down on such a regime. Building up resolve against the high-carbohydrate dogma she keeps hearing is the only hard part about staying on her diet. But she feels and looks wonderful on this eating program.

Tom came to me wanting to lose forty pounds. He started his weight loss program by eating no more than three servings of carbohydrates per day. He lost twenty pounds doing this. But in order to lose the last twenty, he needed to eat nearly zero carbohydrates and take 2 to 3 grams of carnitine per day. He could then achieve his weight goal and keep up with his sports activities. This included thirty miles of cycling every weekend. Interestingly, Tom could not do his cycling if he forgot to take his carnitine. The carnitine was crucial for his body to be able to keep his sports endurance high on this low-carbohydrate diet.

So, there are different amounts of carbohydrates that will suit each person. Learn to experiment and find out how many carbohydrates you feel best on. This is best done with the guidance of an enlightened nutritionist who understands the benefits of modifying carbohydrate intake to suit individual needs.

Another reason to avoid high-carbohydrate diets is that they raise levels of the hormone insulin. When insulin levels are high, carnitine does not work as well in promoting energy and weight loss.

To sum up, some carbohydrates are okay. Too much are, for many, a problem. So enjoy your carbohydrates, in moderation. For most people, that means no more than four servings of carbohydrate-rich foods per day. A serving of carbohydrates is as follows:

➤ 1 fruit
➤ 1 medium whole-grain muffin
➤ ¾ cup whole-grain cereal
➤ 1 small potato or sweet potato
➤ ½ cup cooked brown rice
➤ 1 slice whole-grain or 2 slices diet bread
➤ ½ cup pasta

Top Ten Reasons To Eat Fewer Carbohydrates

❶ *High-carbohydrate diets lower HDL cholesterol and raise triglycerides,* which greatly increases your risk of heart disease.

❷ *Carbohydrates raise insulin,* which makes you fat and increases your risk of type II diabetes.

❸ *A high intake of carbohydrates and sweetened beverages is associated with an increased risk of breast cancer.*[53]

❹ *Carbohydrates eaten in excess raise levels of plasminogen activator inhibitor-1,* which increases risk of heart attacks and strokes.

❺ *Eating too many carbohydrates makes LDL cholesterol smaller and denser,* which in turn raises risk of heart and artery disease.

❻ *Eating a lot of starches and sugars raises levels of blood fats following a meal*—a condition called postprandial lipemia—which is another risk factor for heart disease.

❼ *Eating a lot of starches and sugars can increase the likelihood of a yeast overgrowth, a toxic bowel, and impaired ability of the liver to remove toxic materials from the body,* all of which increase risk of disease.

❽ *Pregnant women who eat diets high in carbohydrates form smaller placentas.*[54] This has ominous implications. The formation of the placenta dictates how well the mother will be able to transfer nutrients to the fetus. Further studies are needed to uncover exactly what the long-term effects of diets high in carbohydrates are on the health of newborns.

➒ A *diet high in grains like wheat will contain phytates that reduce the absorption of valuable nutrients like calcium and zinc.* Such a diet will also increase your exposure to highly allergenic compounds such as gluten, found in wheat, rye, and barley.

➓ *Excessive intake of carbohydrates, especially sugar, will weaken immune function.* Too many carbohydrates will also increase the damage that stress can do to the body,[55] a fact widely appreciated in critical care medicine.

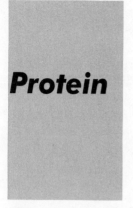

Protein

Do Americans eat enough protein? Some do, some do not. Some eat too much. But for many Americans, particularly women, more protein is needed.

Here is the diet of the average woman who walks into my office:

Breakfast:
Bagel or muffin with coffee

Lunch:
Salad or pasta with minimal protein

Dinner:
Perhaps chicken or fish, rice, and a cooked vegetable and a salad

That is not enough protein for someone to make it through the day with abundant energy. This is a recipe for fatigue.

How much protein do you need? Three to four ounces at each meal is ideal for most people. Some need less, some more. Spreading out your protein intake throughout the day is just as important as getting enough. Eating a twelve-ounce steak at dinner will not benefit you as much as eating four ounces of protein at each meal.

Protein is like oxygen. You cannot just have some at dinner and think you have covered your needs for the day. It's like saying, "I am too busy to breathe this morning. I'll breathe later." You need protein in the morning, at noon, and at dinner. You decide the amount, but don't limit yourself to one protein-containing meal per day like so many do. Doing so limits your health.

PROTEIN SOURCES

Meat, fish, all seafood, chicken, turkey, eggs, cheese, milk

Nuts and Seeds: They contain protein but are still mostly fat. But these fats are beneficial if the nuts are raw. So a small handful of raw nuts per day can be an excellent snack.

Beans/Legumes: These also contain protein, but are mostly carbohydrates. They should be thought of as starches which contain some protein, not primarily as protein foods.

A four ounce serving of meat or fish is the size of a deck of cards.

Dieters in particular need more protein. Those who eat very low-calorie diets have double the protein requirements.[56] Not eating enough protein while dieting causes a loss of muscle tissue. This is undesirable because muscle is where the body burns a lot of fat. Losing muscle slows down your metabolism, so get enough protein at each meal if you are trying to lose weight and keep it off permanently.

According to research done at the USDA, eating enough protein at the end of the day is important for those who want to lose weight and maintain their muscle mass. The body needs protein throughout the night to build and repair itself, and a light evening meal may not give it enough protein to do so. So get adequate protein at every meal, including dinner.

Protein also has 30 to 40 percent more vagus nerve–stimulating ability than carbohydrates or glucose. Stimulating the vagus nerve tells you to stop eating. This is why protein helps curb appetite. This is also one of the reasons it is easier to overeat starches and sugars than protein.[57]

Do not be afraid of protein. There is no reason to be. Those with liver or kidney failure do need to restrict protein intake, but the rest of us can eat protein until we are satisfied. Being afraid of protein is like being afraid of love. It is good for you, and life without an optimal supply of it is just not the same.

THE TEN LAWS OF PROTEIN

Eating optimal amounts of protein is the most important strategy for feeling healthy and keeping your diet in balance. Most people who walk into my office do not eat enough protein. Follow the ten laws of protein, and you will get the most out of its health-building properties:

❶ *Do not fear protein.* It is good for you.

❷ *Protein needs are highly individual.* Science will never fully create a method that will determine how much protein each of us needs for optimal wellness. Experiment. See what amount makes you feel best. This is the best way to determine your individual needs.

❸ *Eat some protein at each meal.* Spreading protein out throughout the day is crucial for you to maximize its benefits.

❹ *Animal protein is superior to vegetable protein.* Vegetable sources of protein can be beneficial, but for protein quality, digestibility, and nutrient content, animal protein rules.

❺ *Protein protects the heart and arteries by raising protective HDL cholesterol.* Many people are afraid of animal protein because they fear it will harm their heart. This is ironic since lean animal protein is one of the most heart-protective foods we have.

❻ *Wild game is the most health-promoting source of animal protein.* When possible, try to consume buffalo, elk, venison, or any game that is harvested from the wild where animals graze freely and are not grain-fed. This creates a much healthier balance of fats in the meat. Cold-water fish such as salmon are also an excellent source of health-promoting protein and beneficial fats.

❼ *Eating protein increases energy and keeps energy balanced throughout the day.* One of the main causes of fatigue in many people, particularly women, is that they are not eating enough protein in the morning and at lunch.

❽ *If you have a lot of sugar and starch cravings, you are not eating enough protein.*

❾ *Stress, exercise, and dieting all increase the need for protein.*

❿ *If you do not digest animal protein well, fix your digestion, don't resign yourself to vegetarianism.* A body that has a tough time digesting meat should not avoid it on those grounds any more than a poorly tuned car should avoid gasoline. Tune up your digestion so that your body can burn the fuel it was meant for! If you have trouble digesting meat, use herbal bitters, hydrochloric acid supplements, and pancreatic enzymes to help you digest meat better. Herbal bitters that contain herbs like gentian are the best place to start. Other digestive supplements are best used under the guidance of a knowledgeable nutritionist.

Top Ten Protein Myths

What are protein requirements? Space does not allow, but a few points could be emphasized. Protein requirements cannot be defined by balance studies. We know that balance can be achieved at any level of intake above some absolute minimum. Whether balance is achieved on a rice diet or a high meat diet— and both obviously occur— tells us nothing about the health of the individuals or the population. We adapt or accommodate to our usual diet. All attempts to define requirements, whether by balance, tissue level, or turnover studies, are really inadequate. The results are affected by the previous diet and experimental design. We do not have a measure of health.

—Mark Hegsted, New England
Regional Primate Research Center,
Harvard University

❶ *If we are in protein balance—a state where the body is not losing any more protein than it is taking in—we are said to be getting all the protein we need.* False. We have to look at other measures as Dr. Hegsted says above. We must look at the overall measure of health. When most of my clients first come to see me, they are eating around 50 grams of protein per day. At that amount, they are not losing muscle mass. But when they increase that to 100 grams per day they feel much better. This is not because they were not in protein balance—they were. But now their protein supply is more optimal and therefore they are healthier If you were given one hundred dollars per week to live on and you could, and that was all you spent, someone might conclude that was all you needed because you were in fiscal balance. But life could be better, even though you could stay in financial balance at that low an amount. Now suppose you were given one thousand dollars per week. You would again be in balance, but the quality of your life would be greatly enhanced. So it is with protein. By looking only at balance studies, we have decided that is the only thing that counts. Nutrition experts use protein to balance blood sugar, promote insulin and female hormonal balance, and to raise beneficial HDL cholesterol. We must therefore think far beyond mere protein balance if we want to find the amount of protein needed for optimal health.

❷ *Eating large amounts of protein from foods such as meat can lower calcium levels in the body and weaken bones.* Not true. Recent research shows that meat-eating does not affect calcium balance.[58] Isolated protein powders may contribute to the loss of bone density,[59] but protein from food such as meat will not cause bone loss.[60] Some studies even suggest that protein promotes stronger bones.[61]

❸ *Beans are basically a protein food.* Partly true but inaccurate. Beans contain protein but are mostly starch. Beans may be an important source of protein for those who cannot afford meat or who are vegetarians. Yet while they do contain more protein than the average vegetable food, beans are mostly starch.

❹ *Protein will damage your liver and kidneys if you eat a lot of it.* Not true. High protein intake is not advised for those with existing liver or kidney disease, but higher protein intake does not cause these conditions. Higher protein and lower carbohydrate intake can help prevent a lot of the ailments that lead to kidney problems such as type II diabetes. Optimal protein intake is also crucial for liver health.

❺ *Soy protein is equal in quality to animal protein.* This is fallacious. Eggs, meat, and dairy products all have superior protein quality compared to soy. Soy is low in the essential amino acid methionine. This limits its ability to promote tissue growth and overall health. Animal studies suggest that whey and meat protein are much more protective against cancer than soy protein.[62] Soy protein has also been found to trigger type I diabetes in animals.[63] I do not recommend soy protein as the chief source of protein in the diet. The only soy foods I recommend are miso, tempeh, and other fermented soy products. These fermented soy foods contain compounds known as isoflavones, which appear to have anticancer effects. Soymilk and tofu do not contain isoflavones in the form that is cancer protective,[64] and soymilk contains phytates that block mineral absorption. Use of soy-based formulas has caused zinc deficiency in infants.[65] Soy protein may lower cholesterol, but it does so in part by lowering beneficial HDL cholesterol.[66]

❻ *Animal protein foods are fattening.* Wrong. Lean meats, eggs, and all high-quality animal products are the best foods for weight loss. Obesity is rare in hunter-gatherer societies that eat only meat and uncultivated vegetables, fruits, and nuts. Obesity is much more common in grain-eating civilizations. In the grain- and carbohydrate-obsessed America of the present, obesity is at epidemic levels.

❼ *We all need the same amount of protein: 0.8 grams per kilogram body weight per day.* Not true. We all have different needs. We will need more protein if we are exercising, have more muscle mass or are under physical, emotional, or mental stress.[67] Illness changes protein needs. Those with HIV or other immune weaknesses need more. Those with Parkinson's disease or autoimmune diseases may benefit from less.

❽ *High-protein diets impair detoxification.* Not usually. Detoxification is the body's process of eliminating metabolic waste before it damages tissues and causes disease. High-protein diets in no way impair detoxification. In fact, they enhance it. In my clinical experience, it is low-protein, high-carbohydrate diets that impair detoxification, because they feed a yeast overgrowth that in turn pushes toxins into the liver and the rest of the body. I find that higher levels of protein—four to six ounces of protein at least twice per day—is essential for a healthy gut and liver and for optimal detoxification. Sulfur-bearing amino acids like methionine, cysteine, and taurine—all crucial for detoxification—are lacking in low-protein and vegetarian diets.

9 *Those who exercise do not need more protein.* They do. The best science we have now suggests that endurance athletes—those who run or do aerobics regularly—should consume 1.4 grams of protein per kilogram body weight. Those who lift weights regularly should consume 1.8 grams per kilogram body weight. This is around twice the current RDA for protein. Athletes have always known they need more protein. Now science is catching up with them.[68]

10 *Protein is toxic because it increases levels of ammonia, which is toxic to the body.* Yes, ammonia is toxic, but a well-nourished body is quite good at turning it into harmless urea. Carnitine found in meat and other animal products helps to quickly detoxify the ammonia that each of us naturally produces in response to a high-protein meal. The toxicity of protein and the ammonia it temporarily generates is greatly exaggerated.

Top Ten Nutrients in Meat

Everyone in health food stores looks pale. Everybody at the
Carnegie Deli looks healthy.

—Jackie Mason

The men's labor was such that each private ate as much as nine
or ten pounds of meat per day.

—Meriwether Lewis's journal, April 27, 1805

A lot of people think meat is bad. Processed meat such as sausages, aged meats, and bologna is not good for you, and meat from animals fed corn and other grains is far from optimal. Meat from grain-fed cattle contains too much of the omega-6 fats—the kinds that can be proinflammatory and procancer when they are not adequately balanced with omega-3 fats.

This does not make all meat bad, however. It only means many of our current versions of meat are bad. If the only time you ever heard Beethoven was when it was played by novices, you might think it bad, but Beethoven is majestic, wonderful stuff, and you will know that only when you hear it played well.

The same is true with meat. The processing of meats and the wrong diet fed to cattle has made meat nutritional cacophony. Let's not judge all meats from looking only at modern processed meats, which do not represent this food fairly. Meats of all kinds can be wonderful for us if the animals are raised and fed correctly. It can be the best food in our diet.

Therefore, everyone should write their meat manufacturers and ask them to feed their cattle flaxmeal mixed in with the grains they are fed. This would give meat a much more healthy balance of fats.

It is very simple and easy to do. This simple act would make an enormous difference in the health of the world. The use of hormones and antibiotics in animal husbandry should also be minimized. These are all realistic goals. If we ask, they will respond to public demand.

Because meat is what we have eaten for most of human history, it should come as no surprise that it can help heal us of allergies to grains and other foods of civilization. A study of 188 children under one year of age who had many food allergies showed that they improved remarkably when fed baby food made of beef heart, broccoli, carrots, and apricots—a diet of just meat and produce. In other words, Paleolithic baby food! Even their formula was made from meat, fruit, and vegetables. The children were allergic to cereal grains, legumes, and milk—foods that humans have not eaten for most of their history. Sixty-two percent of the children had nearly complete relief from their asthma and allergic rhinitis symptoms on this meat and produce diet.[69] A similar Paleolithic diet was used in children with colitis. These children were put on a lamb-based formula, and after two to four days, their symptoms resolved as well.[70]

Is eating meat bad for the environment? While the meat industry does use a great deal of resources to make meat, animals harvested from the wild do not. There are animals that graze on lands that could not support farming. Yes, the commercial meat industry uses a great deal of resources, not the least of which is water, which is a precious commodity in many parts of the world. And there are situations where countries might be better off feeding grains to their starving populations than to animals that are then slaughtered and sold to the well-off.

There is no simple answer to whether meat is good or bad for our environment, because it depends where the meat comes from. Humanity cannot survive without grains, because we do not have the resources for us all to live exclusively on meat. What we need is a balance between meat and grains. It is a balance that the world community will determine as time goes on. But as we continue to determine this balance, we must not use in our discussion the idea that meat is in any way a bad food, because when the animal is raised correctly it is one of the most health-promoting foods we have. Raised in a way that helps the environment, such as animals grazing on unarable lands or those lands currently not under cultivation, meat can be good for the environment as well.

Here, then, are the top ten nutrients in meat:

❶ *Carnitine*, the premier energizing and antiaging nutrient.

❷ *High-quality, nonallergenic protein.* Dairy and grain products are the number-one allergens, which is not surprising when you realize how new they are to the food supply. Humans have eaten meat for hundreds of thousands of years, and very few are allergic to it.

❸ *Omega-3 fatty acids such as EPA and DHA.* They are present in meat when the animals are raised on flaxmeal or forage in the wild.

❹ *CoQ10*, a powerful antioxidant and heart-protecting nutrient found in highest amounts in organ meats.

❺ *Taurine*, a very important amino acid that has unique antioxidant, membrane-stabilizing, and immune-enhancing properties. Vegetarians are particularly susceptible to suboptimal levels of taurine in their diet.

❻ *Zinc*, a crucial nutrient for immune function and brain health. Zinc deficiency is a public health problem in America.[71]

❼ *Carnosine*, a nutrient that acts as a metabolic buffer and one that increases aerobic performance.

❽ *Heme iron*, the best form of iron for building blood. Heme iron is much more beneficial to the body than the synthetic iron found in most supplements. There is also another factor in meat, known as the "MPF factor," which further enhances iron absorption. Meat is also an excellent source for another blood-building nutrient, B_{12}.

❾ *Creatine*, a nutrient that helps build muscle mass and strength.

❿ *Conjugated linoleic acid*, a fatty acid with remarkably powerful anticancer benefits.[72] Conjugated linoleic acid levels are much higher in grass-fed than commerial grain-fed beef.

Another nutrient abundantly found in meat is nucleic acids such as DNA. Nucleic acids like DNA may turn out to be crucial nutrients for the treatment of a range of chronic diseases, and may be another reason why I see health improve in my chronically ill patients when high-quality meat is added back to their diet.[73]

The Fat-Burning Power
of Omega-3 Fats

Wherever flaxseed becomes a regular food item among the people there will be better health.

—Mahatma Gandhi

Now let's take a look at fat, which most people try to avoid. On the surface this seems to make sense, because if we are going to try to get healthy and lose body fat, it seems as though we ought to eat less of it. That may seem right, but that is not the way the body works.

Fat is metabolic. In other words, it does stuff. It influences the metabolism—the sum total of all the activities in your body—with remarkable power. So, if you want to influence your body the right way—promote energy, lose weight, have clear arteries—you need to eat the fats with the most beneficial metabolic effects.

This leads us to inescapably conclude—quite correctly—that it is not *how much* fat you eat that counts. It is *what kind* of fat you eat that determines how healthy you are.[74]

Researchers have assembled a great deal of data to show that getting enough omega-3 fatty acids—those found in flaxseed oil and cold-water fish—is critical for our health. Excessive consumption of omega-6 fatty acids—those found in safflower, sunflower, and corn oils—may be one of the main causes of diseases related to fat consumption.[75] Margarine, shortening, and all junk foods that contain hydrogenated oils should also be avoided, as these fats interfere with omega-3 fatty acids and also greatly increase the risk of heart disease.

So don't just think of fat as something to avoid. Look beyond quantity. Think of quality. If you want to lose weight and be healthy and energetic, use the fats that are going to get you there: omega-3 fats.

There are many reasons flaxseed oil and EPA (an omega-3 fatty acid found in cold-water fish and fish oils) naturally help the body burn fat:

➤ Omega-3 fats increase the activity of carnitine. By so doing, they help the body burn fat better.[76]

➤ Omega-3 fats are burned off more quickly by the body than other fats.

➤ Omega-3 oils are energizing and help you exercise longer.

➤ Flaxseed oil helps the cells of the body—particularly muscle cells—respond more effectively to insulin. This increase in the efficiency of insulin response helps the body burn calories better.

➤ Omega-3 fats like those found in flaxseed oil, consumed early in life, help prevent the development of an excessive number of fat cells. Those with more fat cells are more likely to be overweight. Omega-3 fats can therefore truly be thought of as obesity-preventing fats.[77]

Flaxseed oil is so readily oxidized that it burns off almost as fast as a carbohydrate. It greatly stimulates energy-producing mechanisms in cells. It is so energizing that if you take it before you go to bed, you may have trouble falling asleep.

All of these findings have led many researchers to conclude that flaxseed oil in particular may help prevent and reverse obesity.[78] According to animal studies, alpha-linolenic acid—the name for the omega-3 fat found in flaxseed oil—is burned three times faster in animal studies than stearic acid, a common fat found in animal fats.[79] This has led some researchers to call omega-3 fats "anti-obesity fats."[80] Fish oils have also been found to have a powerful antiobesity effect.[81]

The combination of flaxseed oil with saturated fats yields the most powerful antiobesity effect in animal studies.[82] In other words, it is important to limit the consumption of safflower, sunflower, and corn oils to get the most fat-burning benefits from flaxseed oil. This is because eating other vegetable oils along with flaxseed oil dilutes its metabolic benefits, while eating saturated fats in moderation—those found in butter and coconut oil—does not.

So we have seen that omega-3 fats—those in flaxseed oil, cold water fish, and to a lesser extent in canola oil—help fight obesity in a number of ways. This does not mean you should simply add these oils to your diet, but you should replace the safflower, sunflower, or corn oils with the omega-3 power of flaxseed oil or freshly ground flaxseeds.

DIETING LOWERS OMEGA-3 FATTY ACID LEVELS IN THE BODY

There is another reason why omega-3 fats like flaxseed oil are important during weight loss. When you start to lose weight, omega-3 fats in your body are the first ones to leave.

This is ironic—the most-needed fats are the ones most quickly burned off. Yet they go quickly for a reason: they are the most active fats. That is why it is important to take flaxseed oil—from one teaspoon to many tablespoons per day—throughout your entire weight-loss process.

The whole idea is paradoxical. Eating fat to burn fat. But it works, and is very important for your health as well. You don't want to lose weight and in the process lower your body's level of omega-3 fats, which for most Americans is already too low. You might end up weighing less but also being less healthy. Remember: the goal of weight loss is to get healthy, not merely weigh less. There are plenty of sick thin people. Don't become one of them. Consume plenty of omega-3s fats, especially when you are trying to lose weight.

The omega-3 strategy works. I have seen this time and time again in my clinical practice. I consider flaxseed oil and other omega-3 foods essential for promoting healthy, permanent weight loss. Those who fail to get enough omega-3 fats during weight loss find that they regain their weight easily. They also find they have a tougher time losing weight the next time they try. They have created a lack of omega-3s in their body. This makes their insulin work less effectively and slows their metabolism.

I often see the long-term effects of omega-3 fatty acid deficiency and the resultant slowed metabolism. I see it in people who come

CARNITINE CASE HISTORY

Jennie was a model in New York who was five-foot-eight and weighed 134 pounds when she came to see me. She was under pressure to lose ten pounds so that her agency could book her for more modeling assignments. Her extra weight was mostly around her midsection and hips, and she had difficulty losing this weight even when doing aerobic exercise regularly and eating a low-fat diet. Jennie had a history of eating disorders, so I was careful to help her lose weight in a healthy way that was not too restrictive and that would not create an unhealthy relationship between her and food.

I put her on the Carnitine Program Phase I, 2,000 mg of carnitine per day, a tablespoon of flaxseed oil, 400 mcg of chromium picolinate, and a high-potency multivitamin. She lost between one and two pounds per week, and found the diet easy to follow while eating out, which is where she ate most of her meals. When she got within three pounds of her goal, her weight loss plateaued, so I switched her to the Carnitine Program Phase II and added 1,000 mg of garcinia extract to her supplement program. She reached her weight-loss goal and has maintained it nicely. She looks great and healthy at 124 pounds, a weight I feel genuinely suits her. Every day she takes 1,000 mg of carnitine along with a teaspoon of flaxseed oil, and limits her carbohydrates to keep herself at her new weight.

into my office complaining of difficulty losing weight. For them, low-fat diets do not work, but adding carnitine and flaxseed oil or fish oils to their diet does. Those who understand the metabolism of the body can get it to do what they want. Give your body what it wants to burn fat, and you will get weight loss. If you do not supply the body with the right nutrients, even very low-calorie diets will fail.

Sue is a good example of this. She is a nurse and is overweight. She has tried every diet imaginable. She once ate protein shakes as part of a six hundred calorie per day diet. She lost fifty pounds doing that, but the weight came back slowly over the next year as she returned to her old eating habits. Then she went to one of the diet places that sells you prepackaged food, and lost twenty pounds again. That weight came back eventually as well.

Now Sue is seventy pounds above her ideal weight and is approaching menopause at age forty-four. She finally realizes she needs to work with a health care practitioner who can help her lose weight responsibly, so she seeks the guidance of a dietitian in the hospital where she works. The dietitian earnestly tries to get her to lose weight by putting

Sue on a low-fat, high-carbohydrate diet. The result? Sue gains more weight and gets even more depressed about her weight.

Why does all this happen? Sue has burned off a lot of her omega-3 reserves, which are the first and easiest to burn off, but rarely the ones found in diets, particularly those designed for weight loss. These omega-3s are precisely what she needs to burn fat. She doesn't have them, so fat accumulates in her body. As we have seen, these active fats—the omega-3s in particular—decline after prolonged periods of dieting if they are not generously supplied by the diet.[83] The result? A sluggish metabolism.

Ultra–low fat menus and refined prepared foods like the ones Sue has been on are the worst things you could eat when losing weight. They do not replenish the body with the right fats. Short term, you lose weight. Long term, your metabolism slows and you get fatter.

By eating these mediocre diets, Sue developed a deficiency of omega-3s. Our well-meaning dietitian has implemented a low-fat diet from an essential fatty acid–deficient food pyramid. This further depletes omega-3 fatty acids and Sue gets fatter. The essential fatty acid–deficient food pyramid is creating essential fatty acid–deficient people, especially dieters. The result? A nationwide epidemic of obesity, depression, and heart disease—ailments which are all caused by missing omega-3s.

Weight loss is not merely a matter of calories, but of metabolism. We need to drive our metabolisms with nutrients like omega-3 fats

OMEGA-3s INCREASE NEED FOR ANTIOXIDANTS

When you increase your intake of Omega-3 fats such as flaxseed oil and fish oils, you need to increase your intake of key nutrients which help protect the delicate fatty acids in these foods. You should take at least 400 IUs of vitamin E, or better yet this trio of nutrients:

Vitamin E	400IUs
Vitamin C	500 mg
Selenium	200 mcg

Increasing intake of green leafy vegetables and tomatoes is also recommended to get the boost of all the natural antioxidants found in produce. Or, you could take natural carotenoid supplements with extra lycopene, a powerful carotenoid antioxidant. These nutrients all help protect the delicate omega-3 fats.

and carnitine, not merely starve them with less calories and hope that fat will burn itself off. It may not.

One of the many things that flaxseed oil can do is prevent saturated fats from causing insulin resistance.[84] This is very important, for many of the negative effects of saturated fats are often due to a lack of omega-3s. So, saturated fats are bad for us only when there is a lack of omega-3 fats, or when there is not a good balance between saturated fats and omega-3s, which reminds me of a story. . . .

A FAT STORY

It is very important that a healthy diet should be thought of as a whole rather than as a recitation of good and bad components.

—Michel de Lorgeril

You're on a plane. All of a sudden, you see the flight crew begin to get sick. One by one, the crew begins to become knocked out with food poisoning. Finally, they look for a passenger who can fly the plane. You look calm and collected, so they choose you even though you have no piloting experience.

You crash-land the plane. Everyone lives, but three broken legs are sustained during the evacuation. Pretty good, you think.

A month later, while sitting home, a knock comes at the door. You are being sued by the people with the broken legs. Your crime? "Flying a plane without a license."

What has this got to do with fat? Your omega-3s are the piloting fats. They help promote weight loss, longevity, and protect you against nearly every degenerative disease. When they are not there, passenger fats like saturated fats—innocuous as long as essential fats are in adequate supply—are put into piloting roles they were never meant for. It is not the fault of saturated fats when they falter at doing things other fats were designed for.

So the next time someone blames saturated fats for causing heart disease, just imagine yourself standing at your door served with legal papers. You did your best, but because some other people were not there to do their job, you got blamed. So it is with saturated fats.

For all degenerative diseases, it is what we fail to eat that kills us—especially failing to eat enough omega-3–containing foods.

Omega-3 Dreams

Hearken diligently unto me, and eat ye that which is good, and let your soul delight itself in fatness.

—Isaiah 55:2

Omega-3 fats are so health-promoting and important for disease prevention that if we got more of them, we would reduce the incidence of many diseases. Here, then, are my top ten omega-3 dreams.

❶ *That omega-3 fats will again return to the food supply.* While flaxseed oil and cold-water fish are excellent sources, many people will not eat these foods. We need to have milk, cheese, eggs, meats, muffins, breads, and other main course and snack foods of all kinds incorporating omega-3 fats. This is the only way for the entire population to consume them regularly and reap their benefits.

❷ *That nutritionists organize their education efforts at helping more people include omega-3 fats in their diets.* Omega-3 fatty acids are the number-one nutrient lacking in the American diet and in the diet of many peoples worldwide.

❸ *That America establish a recommended level of intake for omega-3 fats.* Both Canada and England have recommended levels of intake for omega-3 fats—both recommend that people eat these valuable fats at a level of at least 0.5 percent of total calories. That works out to a mere twelve calories as omega-3 fats for someone eating twenty-four hundred calories per day—the amount in one half-teaspoon of flaxseed oil. While this does not seem enough for optimal health, it is at least an acknowledgement of the crucial nature of these fats. Why is it that the American health authorities have not made recommendations regarding the essentiality of these fats? It is time we had at least a five-gram per day recommended intake of omega-3 fats for all Americans.

❹ *That trans fatty acids be listed on food labels.* Trans fatty acids interrupt the function of essential fats in the body, particularly omega-3 fats. Trans fats are found in margarine, shortening, cookies, cakes, cereals, and many other processed foods that list partially hydrogenated or hydrogenated oil as an ingredient. We must have labeling on our foods for trans fats so consumers can know when they are having their fatty acid metabolism harmed and know which foods to avoid.

❺ *That omega-3 content of foods be listed on food labels* so we will know which foods to consume.

❻ *That we realize the importance of the ratio of omega-6 to omega-3 fats in our diet.* Eating too much omega-6 oil causes or accelerates heart disease, cancer, and inflammatory conditions such as asthma and arthritis. We should stop the ad campaigns that have put safflower, sunflower, and corn oils (omega-6 oils) in everyone's cabinet, and stress the need for oils like unrefined walnut, canola, and flaxseed oils, which contain valuable omega-3 fats.

❼ *That the long-chain omega-3 fat DHA be added to infant formula.* DHA is needed by the developing brain, and many countries around the world now add DHA to formula. We should follow their lead. The optimal intelligence and overall mental development of children may be greatly enhanced by this.

❽ *That expecting mothers make sure to consume omega-3 fats at least twice per week throughout their pregnancy*—either in flaxseed or flax oil, purslane, salmon, sardines, or other food sources.

❾ *That omega-3 fats will become routinely used by doctors to treat heart disease, cancer, arthritis, asthma, immune problems, learn-*

ing disabilities, skin disorders, and anything that involves inflam-mation.

🔟 *That fat will again come to be viewed as a mostly good thing.* This is important, for until that happens, we will not come to embrace the goodness of omega-3 fats. They will forever seem in conflict with the "fat is bad" message, which is unfortunately one of the few messages that Americans have successfully received from the nutrition community. We should instead focus our efforts on accentuating the positive, and create an "Omega-3s are good" message.

The Carnitine Program

The Carnitine Program is an eating program that puts together everything we have learned so far. While the Carnitine Program is designed primarily for weight loss, it also forms the nutritional basis for the treatment of a wide range of health problems that we will discuss in the last section of the book.

The Carnitine Program is simple. It is easy to follow because it is built on principles, not rules. It is a flexible, easy way of eating, and you need to think of it as more than merely a series of menu plans.

Menu plans, of course, can be helpful. That's why they are included in this book. But as you work with them, realize two things:

➤ *They are meant to be flexible and changed according to your needs. If you see turkey and want to have chicken or some other meat, make that change. If you do not like the vegetable suggested, eat some other vegetable. Learn the diet in outline form and you will find it easy to make these substitutions.*

➤ *The principles that underlie the menu plans are more important than the menus themselves.*

The principles of the Carnitine Program are the Paleolithic principles we looked at earlier. They should be the principles that guide you in the way you eat for the rest of your life. The four principles at the heart of the Carnitine Program are as follows:

- ➤ Eat protein at each meal.
- ➤ Eat fewer carbohydrates.
- ➤ Eat good fats.
- ➤ Eat whole foods.

That's it. Understand these principles and you have understood the Carnitine Program. If you can do these four things, you will be a lot healthier, you will lose weight, and your cholesterol and triglycerides will be in a good range. This basic, simple strategy has helped hundreds of my clients lose weight and accomplish their health goals. It is so simple! You will feel good on this program, eliminate cravings, and have the energy you need to get through the day.

The only difference in the two phases of the Carnitine Program is the amount of carbohydrates eaten, which is more restricted in Phase II. Otherwise, both phases are very much the same in these four principles.

Now let's look at the two phases of the Carnitine Program in depth.

CARNITINE PROGRAM PHASE I

Phase I of the Carnitine Program allows no more than four servings of carbohydrate-rich foods per day, from a combination of four servings of fruits and/or starches. Proteins can be consumed as needed, and fats need not be counted exactly, as long as they are quality fats and are eaten in moderation. Nonstarchy vegetables such as leafy greens can be eaten freely.

Everyone who wants to lose weight should start with phase I of the Carnitine Program and stay on the diet for two months before assessing whether they need to move to phase II.

CARNITINE PROGRAM PHASE II

Phase II of the Carnitine Program allows zero to one servings of carbohydrates per day. High-quality proteins and fats as well as nonstarchy vegetables may be consumed freely.

Phase II is designed for those who are not losing weight on phase I of the Carnitine Program, and for those with health problems that require more severe carbohydrate restriction, such as very high levels of triglycerides, digestive disturbances, or type II diabetes. Phase II features more marked carbohydrate restriction and is a ketosis-inducing diet.

Phase II of the Carnitine Program—a ketogenic diet—is not appropriate for type I diabetics or pregnant women. These are two groups who should not be in ketosis. It is also not recommended for those with liver or kidney problems. It is safe, however, for nearly everyone else.

Calories in both phases of the Carnitine Program can vary, particularly in phase II. The program can go as low as 1,000 calories, but can also be as high as 2,000 calories or more. I do not recommend going much below 1,000 calories per day, as such low-calorie diets do not work, and also upset carnitine metabolism and thyroid hormone health.[85] So, don't starve yourself. It doesn't work.

The eating strategy I outline below has worked for the vast majority of people I have seen in my practice. It is flexible, and I recommend it as the starting point for most people who want to be healthy.

The Carnitine Program Phase I

Let us look at Phase I of the Carnitine Program in very simple terms:

PROTEIN

2–3 servings per day

Serving sizes:
4–6 ounces of tuna, 1–3 eggs, 5 ounces of fish, 6 medium shrimp,
4 ounces of cheese, 1–2 lamb chops, 4 ounces of any meat (steak,
hamburger, buffalo, elk, venison)

FATS

Use quality fats in moderation

Quality fats: flaxseed oil, virgin olive oil, expeller pressed canola oil
Raw nuts and seeds: almonds, sesame seeds, hazelnuts, and
cashews are best
Acceptable fats: coconut oil, sesame oil, butter
Limit: safflower oil, sunflower oil, corn oil, rice bran oil
Avoid: margarine, hydrogenated and partially hydrogenated oils,
fried foods

VEGETABLES

Eat freely

Arugula, bean sprouts, broccoli, Brussels sprouts, cabbage, cauli-
flower, celery, chicory, collards, cucumber, dandelion greens, eggplant, endive, escarole, green beans, kale, leeks, mushrooms, okra,
parsley, Romaine lettuce, scallions, Swiss chard, water chestnuts

FRUITS

1–2 servings per day

Serving sizes:
1 apple, 3 apricots, 1 cup of any berries, 1 small banana, ¾ cup
cherries, 1 fig (fresh), ½ grapefruit, 1 cup grapes, 1 guava, 2 kiwis,
½ mango, ½ melon, 1 nectarine, 1 orange, ½ papaya, 2 peaches,
1 small pear, ½ persimmon, 3 slices of pineapple, 2 plums,
1 quince, 2 tangerines, 1 cup watermelon

STARCHES

1–2 servings per day

Serving sizes:
½ cup pinto or other beans, ½ cup oatmeal, ½ cup millet, ½ cup
lentils, 1 medium potato, 1 sweet potato, 1 slice whole-grain
bread, 2 slices diet bread

Vegetables that need to be counted as starches:
1 cup carrots, 1 cooked onion, ½ cup peas, ½ cup black-eyed peas,
½ cup corn, 3 cups plain popcorn

**Total servings of fruits and starches: four, with ideally
no more than two coming from the starch category.**

If you understand this outline, you will understand exactly how to do Phase I of the Carnitine Program. You can adjust the serving sizes to suit your own needs. If you are exercising a lot, have a lot of muscle on your frame, or weigh more, you will need more protein and more calories. You may need a fifth serving of fruits or starches per day as well.

Now let's look at more guidelines to help you understand the Carnitine Program.

BREAKFAST

There are two breakfast guidelines:

➤ **Eat some protein.** *This can be eggs, cottage cheese, yogurt, goat cheese, or smoked salmon. But it can also be steak, steak and eggs, chicken, turkey, or anything you enjoy that has protein. Nuts and seeds or nut and seed butters can be excellent when eaten in moderation, particularly when you grind them fresh yourself. The amount is flexible. Experiment.*

➤ **Don't overdo the carbohydrates or sugars.** *One fruit or starch serving with breakfast is fine, but don't make breakfast a carbohydrate festival. Two or three pieces of fruit is not a breakfast that will hold most of us through the morning. We need to balance our morning meal.*

There are many good protein foods to include in your breakfast. For some, eggs, yogurt, and cottage cheese quickly become tiresome. So innovation is in order.

First of all, break the stereotype that breakfast foods cannot include foods traditionally eaten later in the day. I have many clients who are happy to eat salmon, chicken, and other foods for breakfast. One man loved beef stew in the morning. Find what you like to eat that satisfies the two breakfast principles and enjoy it— whether you are eating foods considered "breakfast foods" or not.

One of my favorite recommendations for breakfast is something involving omega-3 oils combined with protein. This usually means flaxseed oil or freshly ground flaxmeal. For ease of digestion, I often recommend that flaxmeal be soaked overnight in water to help make it more digestible.

Note: When adding flaxmeal to shakes, it is recommended that you first grind the flaxmeal before adding any other ingredients to your blender or food processor. If you do not soak your flaxmeal overnight, you will need to add a little bit of water to help your blender or food processor grind up your flaxmeal.

LUNCH

Lunch is often on the go, so it is the meal that requires the most forethought to do well. Preparation is key. Here are some ways of navigating the obstacles of impulsive noontime hunger:

➤ *You can bring leftovers, or think of a place—deli, salad bar, restaurant—that will serve you foods suited the Carnitine Program.*

➤ *Don't be afraid of a chef's salad. Yes, the dressing can have a lot of calories, but hold the croutons and breadsticks and you'll be on track with the Carnitine Program. Ask for the dressing on the side, and be sure to avoid the fat-free dressings. They are loaded with sugar.*

➤ *When eating at a salad bar, get your protein foods first: tuna, beef, chicken, cheese, and then add some garbanzo beans and green vegetables. Don't start with the carbohydrates, or your plate will be full before you get to protein foods.*

DINNER

You need to eat enough protein at dinner so that you can rebuild tissues during the night that need repair after the stress of the day. Don't believe the "eat dinner like a pauper" theory and eat too little at the end of the day. Eat dinner like a person who wants optimal health. This means consuming adequate protein—between three and six ounces for most people.

SNACKS

Some do not feel the need to snack. Others do. Eat according to your needs. Don't be afraid to snack if you need to. Try not to snack, however, more than twice per day.

Snacks on the Carnitine Program should always contain some protein and be balanced with carbohydrates. Don't snack on carrots, popcorn, rice cakes, or fruit by themselves. These carbohydrate snacks do not help the hormonal balance and lean-tissue maintenance we need for weight loss, good energy levels, and good cholesterol levels. Snacks like this will not be filling, because they do not give your body the protein it craves.

Snack ideas:
  - ➤ *One or two small carrots with almond butter*
  - ➤ *Lean chicken, turkey, or roast beef with mustard or other condiment*
  - ➤ *Five to ten raw almonds or cashews with an apple*
  - ➤ *Three to six olives*
  - ➤ *Freshly ground seeds and nuts put on whole-grain crackers (make with organic seeds in coffee grinder— incredible gourmet taste! And fabulous for you.)*

I often recommend late-night snacks of protein foods. I find this very helpful for those with fast metabolisms, and for people of all kinds who are under stress. Before bed, the body is about to embark on eight hours of no food. If you did that during the day, you would not feel well. At night, you need protein to rebuild and maintain tissues. So a small piece of chicken or turkey before bed—especially if dinner was three to five hours ago—is a good idea for many. People who do this often tell me they awake more refreshed and ready for the new day.

For those who do not feel like eating right before bed, but want to help themselves hold on to the muscles they have worked hard to develop when they exercise, I recommend one teaspoon of L-glutamine powder (about 4–5 grams) in a glass of water right before bed. It is a terrific way to help your body stay leaner by keeping muscle tissue optimally nourished.

IMPROVISING ON THE CARNITINE PROGRAM

The best way to do the Carnitine Program is to improvise on it. You will find this easy and fun to do.

Here are ten simple guidelines to help keep you on track as you go through your busy day. Just remember that you need to:

❶ *Eat protein at each meal.*

❷ *Keep carbohydrate intake low.* The amount will differ for each person. Don't be strict all the time. Just remember that carbohydrates are the preferred food for weight gain in the animal industry, and you will see why they are best limited for those who like to be slim.

❸ *Eat according to your hunger.* At times, you may want only a very light meal. At other times, you may want more protein than your menu suggests. Go with your instinct as long as your instinct is for real food, not junk food. Usually, a desire for meat and protein foods is real, while the desire for a candy bar or a Twinkie is a sign of low blood sugar or a yeast overgrowth. Know the difference in the "Simon says" game of food-craving signals, and you will know what your body really wants.

❹ *Eating more than three meals per day is fine if you need it.* Just make sure they are balanced with protein and carbohydrates. An extra-late meal or snack is also fine and helps many lose weight and feel better.

❺ *If you are doing a lot of exercise or are under a lot of stress, you will need more food.* Just make it food that follows the guidelines of the Carnitine Program.

❻ *Do not count calories.* People do not do it in the wild, so you should not do it either.

❼ *Try to get omega-3 fats in your diet where you can.* Flaxseed oil, canola oil, nonfarmed salmon from the wild, sardines, and other cold-water fish are good sources.

❽ *Do your best at restaurants.* Follow the top ten rules for eating out.

❾ *Take a day off the diet now and then and eat what you want.* Make this fun, not restrictive. You should feel good on the diet and enjoy what you are eating.

❿ *Now and then a meal higher in carbohydrates is fine*—the occasional plate of pasta with a sauce, or a vegetarian meal when your macrobiotic friends ask you over. Just realize that if you are in ketosis, this will pull you out of it for a day or so. Such high-carbohydrate meals are more easily done by those following the Carnitine Program Phase I.

If you are still having trouble creating your own diet, or want some professional assistance, call Designs for Health®, a group of cutting-edge nutritionists I have trained to help people achieve a new level of health. Designs for Health refers to the educational institution I run as well as the family of nutritionists who have gone through the training I conduct with Linda Lizotte, R.D. These nutritionists are all accomplished and like-minded in their goal of promoting optimal health. If you have trouble following the suggestions in this book, call the number in the appendix and Designs for Health will direct you to a nutritionist in your area who can help you.

CARNITINE CASE HISTORY

Tim did not like supplements, and wanted to lose weight with diet alone. I accommodated his wishes, and put him on the Carnitine Program Phase I on which he initially he lost one to two pounds per week. After six weeks, he was no longer losing much weight. He was very eager to lose, so I put him on 3,000 mg of carnitine per day—two capsules of 500 mg of carnitine before each meal. After his first week on this regime, he lost five pounds. He then continued to lose at the rate of about two pounds per week until he reached his goal. He felt much more energetic while taking the carnitine, and was thrilled to see the weight finally come off.

TEN TIPS FOR EATING OUT ON THE CARNITINE PROGRAM

❶ *Do not let anyone put rolls, bread, chips, or popcorn on your table while you are ordering.* Elect a bread-basket blocker before you go into the restaurant. Ask if a selection of raw vegetables with a dip is available instead. Those who do well on this eating program are not those with will power; they are those who figure out how to limit their contact with foods they can't resist. Preparations like this are key to following the program successfully.

❷ *Drink water or herbal tea, occasionally wine* if it is something you have as part of your lifestyle. (Alcohol is more bad for you than good. Yes, it can be good for you, but it still damages nerve and liver cells even if it helps our arteries.) No sodas, sugary beverages, or diet sodas. I hate aspartame because of countless clients who have reported everything from headaches to foggy brain function when they ingest it. It's safety is far from established.

❸ *Order a salad with a real dressing, not a sugar-containing fat-free one.*

❹ *Have soups, not starchy appetizers.*

❺ *Ask for meals that are cooked with a variety of spices,* such as garlic, rosemary, oregano, thyme, basil, and ginger. Limit salt intake, but not to zero.

❻ *Have cooked vegetables, not a baked potato,* with your meal.

❼ *Ask for main courses that are broiled, baked, or grilled,* not fried, deep fried, or cooked in a frying pan. Restaurants are very good at making such alterations in the way they cook virtually all of their main-course entrees.

❽ *When eating Italian, try to avoid pasta main courses.* Instead, order meat or seafood dishes. Tell the waiter not to bring pasta as a side dish.

⑨ *Have a gourmet main-course experience so satisfying that you do not want dessert.* Look for your pleasure during the main course, and look not to dessert to rescue you from mediocre cooking, as is so often the case with much of the home cooking in America.

⑩ *Do not be perfect.* If the dessert chef is extraordinary, have something. If you feel like indulging, pick something that is rich tasting but not too sweet, ideally something with chocolate. Chocolate desserts can be wonderful even when minimally sweetened. Chocolate has many protective phenolic compounds that protect our arteries, and fat in chocolate is heart-friendly. Just make such dessert-eating the exception, not the rule.

The Carnitine Program Phase I Menus

To make the foods on these menus, you will need only one extra piece of equipment: a coffee grinder. This will be used for grinding flaxmeal and other items. It is available at most houseware stores for around twenty dollars and is well worth it. To make freshly ground flaxmeal, put the flaxseeds into the coffee grinder and grind for thirty seconds. Shake the grinder a bit while grinding to make sure that the flaxmeal is being evenly ground.

Baked sliced sweet potatoes are a favorite of mine, and I often recommend them with breakfast and dinner. Slice a sweet potato as thin as you can—in a food processor if you have one—and then bake on a cookie sheet for 25 minutes at 300°F. They make the perfect accompaniment to everything from eggs to a hamburger and are loaded with nutrients! Kids love them. Sprinkle with rosemary before cooking for extra flavor and antioxidant activity.

To make flaxseed/olive oil dressing, use ½ flaxseed oil, ½ olive oil, and use your favorite dressing mix. Most people do not notice any taste difference, and this allows you to get more of the fat-burning and health-enhancing power of flaxseed oil into your diet and that of your loved ones.

Sometimes I recommend green tea with breakfast. It is up to you how often you use it. Green tea has some caffeine in it, is mild in taste, and is the most health-promoting beverage for starting your day and for helping weight loss. Put a cinnamon stick in it to flavor it. You can use any other herbal tea or water, but do not use juice regularly in large quantities. Juice has too much sugar in it to be consumed regularly in the Carnitine Program.

ESSENTIAL SUPPLEMENTS FOR CARNITINE PROGRAM PHASE I

Carnitine	1,000–3,000 mg per day in divided doses taken ten minutes before breakfast and lunch
High-potency iron-free multi-vitamin	1–3 per day with meals
Water	6–8 eight-ounce glasses per day

DAY 1

Breakfast

8 ounces sugar-free yogurt or cottage cheese
1 tablespoon flaxseed oil
1 tablespoon fruit preserves or fresh fruit
green tea

Lunch

4 ounces sliced turkey (white meat)
Dijon mustard to taste
2 slices diet bread
large spinach salad with blue cheese dressing

Dinner

1–3 broiled lamb chops with mint jelly
asparagus with hollandaise sauce or butter
1 baked sweet potato
Caesar salad with dressing but no croutons

DAY 2

Breakfast

¾ cup cooked oatmeal
3 tablespoons freshly ground flaxmeal
2 tablespoons organic raisins
¼ teaspoon cinnamon

Lunch

tuna-salad sandwich with mayonnaise, chopped celery, and onion
2 leafs of Romaine or other deep-green lettuce
2 slices diet bread
1 peach or other fruit

Dinner

6 large stir-fried shrimp or 10 scallops with snow pea pods, onions,
bean sprouts, water chestnuts, and broccoli
dipping sauce if desired

DAY 3

Breakfast

¼ cup uncooked oatmeal ground in coffee grinder for one minute
8 ounces goat's or skimmed milk
1 tablespoon flaxseed oil
1 banana
optional: ¼ teaspoon almond extract

*Blend all ingredients in a blender on high speed for one minute.
Crushed ice and/or 2 tablespoons cocoa or carob powder may be
added if flavor is desired.*

Lunch

4–6 oz. crabmeat
1 tablespoon sugar-free mayonnaise
chopped celery
Romaine lettuce with 2 tablespoons gorgonzola cheese or dressing

Dinner

5 ounces grilled or broiled swordfish
butter or pesto sauce (olive/flaxseed oil, pine nuts, basil, garlic, and parmesan cheese)
1 small baked or grilled potato
leafy green salad with dressing

DAY 4

Breakfast

8 ounces cottage cheese
1 tablespoon flaxseed oil
2 tablespoons chopped walnuts or slivered almonds
½ cup berries or other chopped fruit
green tea

Lunch

4–6-ounce hamburger cooked well done, made with lean ground round from antibiotic-free beef such as Coleman's Beef, without bun
1 teaspoon of ketchup or relish
sugar-free condiments such as mustard, salsa, or San J Szechuan sauce may be used freely
2 dill pickle spears
lettuce, tomato, and onion
½ cup sauerkraut
½ cup cole slaw

Dinner

3–6 slices lean London broil
1 pat butter
creamed spinach
green salad with any sugar-free dressing

DAY 5

Breakfast

2–3 ounces warmed goat cheese or other cheese
1 sliced baked apple with cinnamon or one piece raw fruit
green tea

Lunch

4 ounces sliced roast beef or sliced steak
lettuce and tomato
Dijon mustard to taste
2 slices diet bread
1 dill pickle
1 apple or other fruit

Dinner

4–8 ounces of breast of duck or other meat
grilled vegetables: zucchini, onions, potatoes, eggplant
salad with flaxseed oil dressing

DAY 6

Breakfast

2-3 egg omelet with chopped green pepper and onions
sliced baked sweet potatoes with rosemary
green tea

Lunch

4–6 large grilled shrimp
1 bowl vegetable soup
sliced tomato and onions with olive oil and fresh basil

Dinner

4–6 ounces buffalo steak or other lean meat
grilled zucchini
1 small baked potato
1 tablespoon sour cream
Salad with flaxseed/olive oil dressing

DAY 7

Breakfast

1 cup regular Cheerios
8 ounces skimmed milk or, better still, goat's milk
½ cup fresh berries

Lunch

Chef's salad
Gorgonzola, blue cheese, mayonnaise, or any dressing desired

Dinner

4–8 ounces organic chicken or Cornish game hen
Steamed broccoli with hollandaise sauce
Green salad with dressing

SNACKS FOR PHASE I
OF THE CARNITINE PROGRAM

Have zero to two snacks per day, according to your needs.

hard boiled egg, Neufchatel cheese on celery stick, five macadamia nuts, two tablespoons raw sesame seeds, three to six olives, two ounces lean meat with mustard, small handful almonds or other raw nuts, roasted garlic or almond butter on a rice cracker or a Wasa rye cracker

The Carnitine Program
Phase II: The Ketogenic Diet

Ketone bodies are a source of fuel for the body and function in the same way as glucose and fatty acids.

—*Nutrition: An Integrated Approach,*
Pike and Brown, 1984, p. 525

I have a friend who lives in Vancouver. He loves it. He jokingly said I should tell people it is not that great a place to live. "Why?" I asked. "So people will stop moving here."

That is the only explanation I can have for the message one hears from certain corners of the nutrition community that says that ketosis is bad. Bad for whom? People who sell diet drugs? Ketosis works. For many people it is very good. It helps people lose weight who otherwise cannot, even on low-fat diets or moderately low carbohydrate diets like the Carnitine Program Phase I.

When you eat very few or no carbohydrates, you push your body into ketosis, a state in which your body burns fat in a unique way. Ketosis gets its name from a group of three compounds called ketone bodies, which are formed during low carbohydrate intake. The body uses these ketones safely and effectively for energy.

Ketone bodies are special fatlike compounds that are water-soluble. They are used for energy by all tissues in the body except the liver. They are a perfectly normal constituent of your metabolism.

Ketosis and ketone bodies play many valuable roles in the body. The heart is constantly using ketone bodies for energy. They have a range of benefits we are only beginning to understand. Ketones may have unique advantages for those who are being fed intravenously.[86]

Ketosis is not recommended for type I diabetics, for those with kidney failure, or for pregnant women. The rest of us can do just fine in ketosis. Tens of thousands of Americans go into ketosis each year with no ill effects, and lose plenty of weight on ketosis-inducing diets. Children with epilepsy go on ketosis-inducing diets and their seizures stop. Long-term studies show that staying in ketosis for years has no adverse effects, and for epileptics in particular has many benefits.[87]

KETOSIS HELPS CERTAIN CANCERS

Ketogenic diets have also achieved impressive results in the treatment of certain cancers, especially those involving the central nervous system.88 Astrocytoma tumors have disappeared in patients who used ketogenic diets incorporating medium-chain triglyceride supplements as 60 percent of the diet. These tumors cannot use ketones for fuel, while body cells can. The ketogenic diet thus starves the tumors by cutting down their uptake of blood sugar. This thwarts their growth.89 While more research is needed, it seems for those patients with astrocytoma tumors and other cancers in the nervous system, the ketogenic diet is worth a try.

KETOSIS IS SAFE FOR ATHLETES

A recent study showed the safety of a ketosis-inducing diet. Five trained athletes went on a low-carbohydrate diet for four weeks. On this diet, most of their calories came from fat. After being in ketosis for four weeks, their aerobic endurance was tested. In ketosis, they had the same aerobic endurance after four weeks of ketosis as they did on a mixed diet with plenty of carbohydrates. They used fat just as well as carbohydrates as their energy source, and the ketosis diet had no ill effects on their health or sports performance.[90]

APPROACH KETOSIS GRADUALLY

I do not recommend that people go into ketosis without first trying the Carnitine Program Phase I. Not everyone needs to be in ketosis to lose weight, conquer yeast overgrowth, or deal with other problems related to carbohydrate intake. But some do, and for them, a very low carbohydrate diet that leads to ketosis will be the only answer.

CARNITINE CASE HISTORY

Jennie came to me in March wanting to lose weight in time for a Fourth of July boat party, where she wanted to display a new, slimmer figure. In less than four months, she wanted to lose thirty-five pounds. I put her on the Carnitine Program Phase I for the first two months, along with 2,000 mg of carnitine per day and a high-potency multivitamin, and she lost weight at a pace of between one and two pounds per week. By May, we still had eighteen pounds to go, so I increased her carnitine to 3,000 mg per day and put her on the Carnitine Program Phase II. She made her weight loss goal in time and was pleased with her diet and supplements, and proud of the new, slim physique she had created for herself.

You should ideally be checked for any preexisting kidney problems before going on a very low-carbohydrate diet. Anyone with any history of kidney weakness should not go into ketosis and should have their nutrition needs monitored by a physician and/or nutritionist who specializes in kidney health.

The ketogenic diet should also be, where possible, one that emphasizes quality fats, especially omega-3 fats and medium-chain triglycerides. Nutrients such as carnitine and CoQ10, as well as all the antioxidants, are essential for helping the body deal with the rapid weight loss seen in ketosis.

Carnitine is especially important for ketosis, for it helps the liver make blood sugar from protein in the diet, a process called gluconeogenesis. This all but eliminates any fatigue or headaches that sometimes can occur in ketosis. It is a shame that everyone who goes into ketosis does not use high-quality carnitine supplements. This would eliminate the fatigue that often forces them to go off a ketogenic diet. All they are missing is the carnitine! Carnitine is not a pair of fuzzy dice hanging from the rear-view mirror—it is the nutritional engine that drives the power of low-carbohydrate living. Carnitine ensures that energy levels will be kept high by helping the body make the adjustment from burning predominantly carbohydrates to burning fat for energy.[91]

If you have tried carbohydrate restriction in Phase I of the Carnitine Program and it has not worked, move on to phase II, the ketogenic diet. Popularized by Robert Atkins, M.D., this diet has been one of the most valuable clinical tools I have used over the many years of my practice.

The menus below are meant to be modular, and any substitutions of meats for other proteins can be made. The only rule is to avoid the following foods completely: Bread and bread products (rolls, breadsticks, etc.), sugar, fruit, candy, pasta, oatmeal, and all those foods that are high in carbohydrates.

The ketogenic diet as done in phase II of the Carnitine Program is very similar to the Paleolithic diet for all people who lived above 40° latitude and for those who lived in temperate zones during the winter months.. It is one where legumes and grain products are limited, and mainly animal products and fruits and vegetables are eaten. No wonder so many people do well on it: it is the diet their body has eaten for millions of years.

Carnitine Program Phase II Menus

The key to enjoying the Carnitine Program Phase II is not to worry about the exactness of your serving size. The only thing you need to do is keep carbohydrate intake as low as possible, eat protein at each meal, and emphasize healthful fats where possible. Eat until you are satisfied!

ESSENTIALSUPPLEMENTS FOR CARNITINE PROGRAM PHASE II

Carnitine	1,000–4,000 mg per day in divided doses before breakfast and lunch
MCT oil	1 tablespoon per day with breakfast
High-potency iron-free multi-vitamin	1–3 per day with meals
Fiber supplement	1 tablespoon with 8 ounces water, 1–3 times per day 20 minutes before meals
Water	6–8 eight-ounce glasses per day

Call 1 (800) USE-FLAX to get pure MCT oil from Allergy Resources if you can't find it in your health food store. The best fiber supplement is flaxmeal fiber from Omega Nutrition, available in health food stores or by calling 1 (800) 661-3529. Even better, get flaxseeds and grind them yourself fresh daily in a coffee or seed grinder. Psyllium powder or other fiber blends can also be used, but they have nowhere near the health benefits of flaxmeal powder.

Drinking six to eight glasses of water per day is especially important during the Carnitine Program Phase II. The body needs plenty of water when protein intake is high, and especially during ketosis. Do your best to get as close to eight glasses of water per day as you can. You may drink more if desired. Don't wait for thirst to prompt you, for you often need more water than thirst will indicate when in ketosis.

DAY 1

Breakfast

1 cup cottage cheese or eight ounces of yogurt with no sugar added
1 small handful chopped nuts
1 tablespoon flaxseed oil
1 teaspoon fructooligosaccharides syrup (FOS)—*available in health food stores*

Lunch

3–6 slices turkey (white meat) or any selection of meats and cheeses
spinach salad
blue cheese dressing or any other sugar-free dressing

Dinner

1–3 broiled lamb chops
asparagus with hollandaise sauce
Caesar salad with dressing but no croutons

DAY 2

Breakfast

2 slices lean ham with 1–2 slices melted cheese
2 Wasa 25-calorie rye crackers
green tea

Lunch

1 six-ounce can of tuna
2 tablespoons mayonnaise or pesto sauce
chopped raw carrots and celery

Dinner

stir-fried shrimp or scallops with snow pea pods, onions, bean
sprouts, broccoli

DAY 3

Breakfast

any selection of cheeses (Jarlsburg, cheddar, goat)
½ sliced cucumber
green tea

Lunch

4–6 ounces crabmeat
1–2 tablespoons mayonnaise
chopped celery
Romaine lettuce with gorgonzola

Dinner

grilled swordfish with Cajun spices
2 pats butter
large leafy green salad with dressing

DAY 4

Breakfast

cottage cheese or yogurt with no sugar added
1 tablespoon flaxseed oil
chopped walnuts
green tea

Lunch

Chef's salad with any dressing desired

Dinner

4–6 slices London broil
1 pat butter
1 cup steamed broccoli
creamed spinach

DAY 5

Breakfast

warmed goat cheese
sliced ripe tomatoes
green tea

Lunch

deviled eggs
French onion soup
sautéed greens in garlic and olive oil

Dinner

breast of duck
grilled zucchini
salad with flaxseed/olive oil dressing

DAY 6

Breakfast

2–3-egg omelet with chopped bell pepper, mushrooms, and onions
2 tablespoons salsa
green tea

Lunch

grilled shrimp or other seafood
vegetable soup
sliced tomato and onions with fresh basil and olive oil

Dinner

buffalo steak or any lean meat
1 cup grilled vegetables
arugula salad with flaxseed/olive oil dressing

DAY 7

Breakfast

2–3-egg omelet
1–2 ounces smoked salmon
2 Wasa 25-calorie rye crackers
green tea

Lunch

4–6-ounce hamburger without bun made with lean ground round
from antibiotic-free beef such as Coleman's Beef
1 teaspoon of ketchup or relish
sugar-free condiments such as mustard or salsa may be used freely
2 dill pickle spears, lettuce, tomato, and onion
½ cup sauerkraut and ½ cup cole slaw

Dinner

Cornish game hen
steamed broccoli with hollandaise sauce
green salad with flaxseed/olive oil dressing

hard boiled egg, any cheeses, small handful of nuts, three to six olives, two sun-dried tomatoes in olive oil, Neufchatel cheese on celery stick, five raw macadamia nuts, two tablespoons raw sesame seeds, any meat with mustard or some other sugar-free condiment

For variations with above menus, substitute any meat or fish-based food anywhere you like. As long as you avoid carbohydrate foods completely, you can basically do anything you like!

TRANSITIONING OFF PHASES I AND II
OF THE CARNITINE PROGRAM

After you have achieved your weight-loss goals, you can begin to add carbohydrates back to your diet. Carbohydrates are your accelerator, and your brake. When you want to lose weight, remove them as much as is needed for you to get to your goal. When you are at the weight you want to be, add them back—slowly.

I generally recommend adding one carbohydrate back per day every week until you see how you feel. Don't go carbohydrate crazy, though, or you will find yourself back where you started from. The most difficult part of keeping weight off long-term is respecting the fattening power of excess carbohydrates. Respect it.

SUPER-HEALTHY LOW-CARBOHYDRATE FOODS

If you are not acquainted with all of these foods, you should be. They make the Carnitine Program very easy and enjoyable to follow.

Olives

Snacking on olives is a great way to enjoy yourself on the Carnitine Program. A few years ago a nutrition newsletter warned about the dangers of olives because they are "high in fat." That is precisely what is good about them. They are high in a healthful fatty acid, oleic acid, that has benefits on blood sugar and insulin metabolism, as well as a range of other health-promoting compounds.

Nuts and Seeds

Nuts and seeds are the most concentrated source of nutrition you can find in food. They are extraordinarily high in minerals, and studies show that those who eat nuts regularly are slimmer and better protected against heart disease. They do contain some carbohydrates, so have only a small handful per day if you are on the Carnitine Program.

Cheeses

Try to find cheeses that are high in omega-3 fats. This will be difficult, but if animals are fed flaxmeal and grasses instead of grains, then the cheese from their milk will be high in omega-3s as well.

Oils

Flaxseed oil, olive oil, coconut oil, and sesame oil all have health benefits. Gourmet oils such as the delicious pistachio oil (available from Omega Nutrition) are also excellent in taste and nutritional value. Adding them to dishes increases your intake of health-promoting fats. This allows you to get more calories from healthy fats and less from carbohydrates. This is desirable not only for weight loss but for lowered cholesterol and triglyceride readings.

Sauces

Don't be afraid of sauces. As part of a low-carbohydrate diet, they are health-promoting and will help you stay on the diet that will healthfully promote weight loss and better blood cholesterol levels. Hollandaise sauce is loaded with liver-protective phosphatidyl choline. It does contain cholesterol and saturated fats, but studies suggest that you can eat these as part of a healthy diet without raising cholesterol.[92] Pesto sauce made with extra virgin olive oil is loaded with antioxidants. Sauces give you satiety, and help give you a nutrient so often missing in diets: pleasure.

Common Questions about the Carnitine Program

How do I know how much to eat when portion sizes are not listed?

Trust your hunger. When it comes to protein foods, we should eat enough of them to feel satisfied. Our protein needs are all so different that it is a misstatement for anyone to say that protein needs for everyone have been worked out to some magical number or percentage of calories. Protein intake that leads to optimal health differs from person to person. Even those with the same weight and activity level can have dramatically different protein requirements. Most do well on three to six ounces of protein at each meal, but you may do better on more—or less. Experiment and see how you feel.

Regarding carbohydrates—grains, fruits, starchy vegetables—how do you know when you have had enough of these? This is harder, which is why I have listed serving sizes for them. When you do not eat enough protein, you can easily overeat carbohydrates, searching for the protein you need but will not find there. While you can be free with protein, limit yourself to the amount of carbohydrates suggested, for they are easily overeaten.

Salad dressings should be applied reasonably. Salads can be eaten freely, even with dressings. If you keep your carbohydrate intake under control, the amount of fat in salad dressings will not contribute to weight gain, and salad dressings made with flaxseed oil will actually help the weight-loss process.

The goal of the Carnitine Program is to satisfy you on a reasonable amount of food, and to leave you in control of portion sizes as much as possible. The satiety which comes from giving the body the food it needs is the best way to control your food intake. This sets up a healthy relationship between you and food for the rest of your life, for it allows you to be in control of what you eat as you listen to your body and give it what it wants.

Why can't I eat a muffin for breakfast?

Most muffins do not work on the Carnitine Program. The only exception is muffins made with significant quantities of fresh flaxmeal, which are sometimes available at health food stores. But muffins from commercial bakeries and even many health food stores are usually too high in carbohydrates and too low in protein to serve as a healthy breakfast.

Can I drink coffee?

Yes, if you like, but I am not a big fan of coffee. Coffee has some good compounds, but also many health-robbing compounds. I am much more impressed with green tea, which has a wide range of benefits to the heart, arteries, liver, and immune system. If you do insist on coffee, get organic coffee at a health food store if at all possible. Do not put sugar in your coffee. Cream is fine.

I have heard that shrimp are high in cholesterol. Is it okay to eat them regularly?

Shrimp have very beneficial effects on blood cholesterol and triglyceride levels.[93] Do your best to get them from a clean source. Then they are perfectly safe to eat every day.

You recommend nut butters. Aren't they high in fat?

Yes, but their fats are beneficial as long as they are freshly made. I especially like almond butter from raw, not roasted, almonds. Do your best to get nut butters from companies like Walnut Acres—reach them at 1 (800) 433-3998—that make nut butters from organic nuts and make them in small batches. Nut butters should be kept refrigerated and used promptly.

The ideal way to eat nut butters is to buy fresh organic nuts from Walnut Acres or a similar high-quality source and grind them yourself. The coffee grinder I recommend for grinding flaxseeds is also excellent for making nuts butters in small amounts.

I prefer almond butter to peanut butter, but if you do insist on peanut butter, make sure it comes from a company that can guarantee their peanuts do not contain the carcinogenic mold aflatoxin. This is a problem with peanuts, which are grown in very moist environments. Walnut Acres tests their peanuts for aflatoxin. Read labels and write your favorite manufacturer of peanut butter to make sure they are doing the same.

Those who regularly consume nut butters have an increased need for vitamin E, and should take 400 IUs of vitamin E per day.

I am still not comfortable with eating meat every day. Are you sure it is all right?

Yes. Just remember to eat real meat—roast beef, steak, and wild game if at all possible. Try to get your meat from cattle ranchers who treat their animals responsibly, and ideally from those who let their animals graze on grasses or feed them flaxmeal. This will not always be possible, but do your best. Remember, the men of the Lewis and Clark team ate nine to ten pounds of meat each day and enjoyed excellent health. Therefore, you should not be afraid to eat eight to twelve ounces of lean meat during the course of the day. If you want to be afraid of something, be afraid of margarine and too many sugars and starches—this is what causes most of my clients to gain weight, feel tired, and even get depressed. It will take you many months, maybe even years, to learn once again that meat is good. It took me eleven years of vegetarianism to learn it.

When can I eat pasta?

When you want to decrease the quality of your diet. You can take a day or two off the Carnitine Program and have pasta if you really enjoy it. Realize, however, that I and a growing cadre of nutritionists are not convinced that pasta—especially the white-flour pastas that predominate—is anything more than junk food. Yes, pasta is low in fat, but so is gasoline and you don't eat that. Eat food for what it has—not for what it doesn't have—if you want to promote your health. What pasta has is a lot of empty carbohydrates, not much fiber, and a deficiency of protein, which your body so desperately needs to be healthy.

I am tired of drinking water with meals. Can I drink fruit juice?

If you must have fruit juice, dilute your fruit juice with water. Some fruit juice is okay on the Carnitine Program Phase I, but it has too many carbohydrates for the Carnitine Program Phase II. Instead of fruit juice, try squeezing a fresh lemon or lime into your water. If you must have fruit juice, purple grape juice may be the most health-promoting kind. It has the same compounds found in wine that protect our heart and arteries and without all the neurotoxic alcohol.[94] Purple grapes as a snack would be even better. Fruit has so much more to offer than juice and fruit juice is easily overconsumed. I once had a twelve-year-old boy who was twenty-five pounds overweight. He was drinking six glasses of fruit juice per day on top of his regular diet. Eliminating the fruit juice let him lose twenty-five pounds in six months, much to his delight and that of his parents. Once again, the fattening power of carbohydrates—especially refined carbohydrates like sugary fruit juice—easily escapes us.

Better than fruit juice is a fun herbal drink line made by Celestial Seasonings called "Iced Delight." You make it simply by steeping bags of the mix in a pitcher of water in your fridge. They are available in health food stores. I particularly like their Cranberry Razz. These are virtually calorie-free herbal drinks that are easy to make and delicious. You will never drink plain water again.

Can I have drinks sweetened with aspartame?

No. I do not like aspartame. Aspartame-sweetened beverages stimulate people to overeat even more than sugar-sweetened beverages do.[95] I am very worried about its long-term effects on human brain function, which are completely unknown at this time. I feel cloudy-headed when I eat aspartame. When I asked listeners of my nationally syndicated radio show to call in with their feedback on aspartame, I heard horror stories of headaches, seizures, vision disturbances, and other health problems. Do these problems affect everyone? No, but let's wait until it really is proven safe.

Which fats do you recommend cooking with?

The most stable fat for all forms of cooking is coconut oil. Contrary to popular belief, coconut oil has many benefits, may be antiviral as well as anticancer, and does not raise cholesterol levels or contribute to heart disease.[96] Cooking with coconut oil is much better for you than overheating vegetable oils like safflower, sunflower, and corn oils. Overheating these vegetable oils creates dangerous compounds that damage the body. Heating coconut oil does not create problems. Populations that eat a lot of coconut and coconut oil have very low rates of heart disease.[97] Use coconut oil that is organic and unhydrogenated. You can get high-quality coconut oil as well as flaxseed oil from Omega Nutrition at 1 (800) 661-3529.

You say eat yogurt that has no sugar added.
But I read the label and all yogurts contain sugars.

All yogurt has sugars that are naturally present; and when they are listed on the nutritional contents panel of the container, it can make things confusing. What you want to look for is a yogurt with no *added* sugars. Avoid those made with sucrose, high fructose corn syrup, or fruit juice concentrate. Once in a while they are okay, however, don't let them become a habit. It is far better to add fresh fruit to yogurt, like berries or organic raisins. Raisins really must be organic because pesticides put on grapes are very nasty ones indeed.

If you can, I recommend making your own yogurt at home. I do this often and the taste is extraordinary—tangy and delicious. The best part about making your own yogurt is that you have much more control over the quality of the beneficial bacteria present in the yogurt. The bacteria in store-bought yogurts is usually good but not as health promoting as possible. Making yogurt with a yogurt starter made by Natren, however, gives you a very high quality strain of beneficial bacteria called bulgaricus, which has many proven health benefits. Making your own yogurt with fresh goat's milk, if available, is ideal. Natren yogurt starter is available in health food stores or by calling 1 (800) 992-3323.

*When you say cottage cheese for breakfast,
is that regular full-fat, low-fat, or fat-free?*

Low-fat is fine, but you can have full-fat if you desire. Fat-free cottage cheese tastes like wallpaper paste. I do suggest fat-free skimmed milk, however, for those who drink milk, because it will have the lowest levels of xanthine oxidase, a harmful compound found in homogenized milk. If you can get raw certified milk where you are, that is best, and you can drink that whole.

Do I have to take carnitine to lose weight on these menu plans?

No, but it is highly recommended that you do. Carnitine will keep your energy high, help cut cravings, and maximize the amount of weight you will lose. You can lose weight on these plans without carnitine, but it will not happen as quickly.

Is carnitine addictive?

No. You will like the natural energy you feel on carnitine, and will want to experience it on a daily basis, but it is in no way addictive. Heart patients who are taking carnitine, however, should not suddenly stop taking carnitine without talking to their physician, as their heart may need the constant dosing of carnitine for optimal heart function.

*If I take carnitine to help me lose weight,
will the weight come back after I stop taking the carnitine?*

No. Not unless you return to your former eating habits. Carnitine helps weight loss, but you must also eat a health-promoting diet—preferably low in carbohydrates—if you expect carnitine to help you.

How do I know whether to take carnitine or acetyl-L-carnitine?

For weight loss and sports endurance, carnitine is fine. For maximizing brain health, acetyl-L-carnitine is the preferred form. For those over forty, I recommend taking both whenever possible. The only drawback of the acetyl-L-carnitine form is that it is more expensive. Otherwise I would recommend it for everyone.

When will I start feeling the benefits of carnitine?

You should begin to feel an increase in energy within the first few days. If after a week you feel nothing, you may not be taking enough, or you may be taking an inferior brand that may not be delivering what their label claims.

For endurance athletes, it may take a few weeks to a few months of taking carnitine to feel the benefits in sports performance. Heart patients as well should give carnitine therapy a minimum of twelve weeks before they and their physician assess whether it is helping their angina, cardiomyopathy, or other heart problem.

What is the difference between L-carnitine and DL-carnitine?

L-Carnitine is the natural form of carnitine. Only consume L-Carnitine, never D-carnitine or DL-carnitine. These forms are not available in America, because the D-carnitine molecule interferes with the action of the natural L-carnitine.[98]

I am a vegetarian. I know that carnitine is a nutrient found in meat. Are carnitine supplements made from meat or from animal products in any way?

No. If carnitine supplements came from meat they would be incredibly expensive! All carnitine supplements are synthetically made and are suitable for the strictest vegetarians so long as none of the binders or flow agents used in making the carnitine are derived from animal products (they usually are not). Do keep in mind, however, that capsules are derived from animal gelatin. There are, however, new vegetable-derived gelatin capsules that are becoming increasingly popular.

What is the upper limit for carnitine dosing?

I have seen people take up to 4 grams (4,000 mg) of carnitine per day with only positive results. There have been studies that have used doses of up to 15 grams with the only side effect at such high doses being mild, transient diarrhea. Such high doses of carnitine should be taken in divided doses throughout the day. Another side effect of such high doses may make it hard for you to fall asleep. Just remember that carnitine is like vitamin C, and that when taking higher doses, you need to build up your intake slowly so that your body can begin to adjust to the higher doses.

Can carnitine be taken safely with other medications?

Yes, with the caveat that carnitine supports heart function, and that heart-supporting medications may be needed in lower doses when carnitine is used. Heart patients and those with any serious illness should ideally only take carnitine with the supervision of their physician. Carnitine is listed in the *Physician's Desk Reference* for those who want to review its safety data.

Should carnitine be taken with other nutrients?

Yes. When taking it for heart problems, combining it with CoQ10, magnesium, taurine, and vitamin E, for example, is highly recommended. When treating any health problem, taking carnitine with the nutrients outlined in the final section of this book is advantageous. Remember that health problems should always be treated with the guidance of a health care practitioner.

How safe is L-Carnitine?

Extremely safe. Carnitine is so safe that no one has ever overdosed on it or shown any toxicity from taking it, according to the *Physician's Desk Reference.*

Troubleshooting

Why do you seek more knowledge when you do not pay attention to what you already know?

—Zen saying

The main problem with those who are not getting results on the Carnitine Program—be it weight loss or lower cholesterol—usually comes from eating too many carbohydrates. Many clients come to see me, get excellent results with weight loss and cholesterol optimizing, and yet often call me in six months to say that weight is creeping back or blood-lipid levels are back up. The problem is twofold:

➤ The unending propaganda that high-carbohydrate foods are best for you (fallacious)

➤ The ubiquitous nature of carbohydrate foods (muffins, bagels, pasta, bread, cookies, candy, pastries)

The strategy? Become aware of the carbohydrates in your life. Limit them. Make sure you are getting enough protein. That will solve the problems for over 80 percent of those who are not losing weight on the Carnitine Program.

Sometimes the body stops losing weight, even when you do limit carbohydrates. Here is what you can do to get things going again:

TAKE MORE CARNITINE

Sometimes I do not see results with carnitine unless people take 2,000 mg per day, and some people really start to do well only on 3,000–4,000 mg. Increase your dosage of carnitine by 500 mg per day until you start to feel an optimal energy level. This is the sign that your body is finally starting to burn more fat.

USE GARCINIA AND CHROMIUM PICOLINATE WITH CARNITINE

Garcinia extract (Brindall berry) along with carnitine and chromium picolinate has been shown in one study to promote weight loss. I have seen some people benefit from this combination, and all three of these compounds together are perfectly safe to take over the long term. Use 200–400 mcg of chromium picolinate, at least 1,000–2,000 mg of carnitine, and 500–2,000 mg of garcinia extract. This should be combined with the Carnitine Program. Stay on this for one month before you assess whether it is working more effectively than carnitine alone.

FOCUS YOUR FATS

Use just animal fats and omega-3 fats, and pay special attention to avoiding omega-6 fats (safflower, sunflower, corn, rice bran oil). This means using flaxseed oil and neutral oils like olive oil. This strategy has helped many of my clients. We need omega-3 fats like those in flaxseed oil to lose weight, and many people need to strictly avoid the omega-6s if the omega-3s are going to be beneficial.

EXERCISE

Perhaps it is time you finally got moving. Strength training in particular is my favorite exercise for weight loss.[99] Even half an hour of lifting weights three times per week can make a big difference. Ideally, work with a personal trainer or someone at the gym who can motivate you and show you how to do it right. Combining strength training with aerobics and stretching exercises is ideal.

FOOD ALLERGIES

Food allergies can slow down weight loss, further proof that weight loss involves a lot more than counting calories. Consider having a blood test for food allergies to help you pinpoint problem foods. Common food allegies involve grains, dairy products, and yeast, so before spending money on an expensive blood test, try avoiding these foods. I have seen dramatic weight loss in a few cases where people were allergic to unusual foods (tomatoes, for example), and only a blood test was able to determine this.

Acetyl-L-Carnitine and Brain Nutrition

We will now look at a special form of carnitine known as acetyl-L-carnitine, which has a dramatic ability to promote brain wellness.

Brain Nutrition

You are as young as your brain.

—Gernot Treush

We have an enormous amount of influence over the health and function of our brains. The brain is remarkably responsive to what we eat, what we think, and our overall state of health. That's the good news. The bad news is that a lot of what we do damages our brains. Stress, missing nutrients, toxins in our environment and body, and alcohol are the prime offenders. But optimal nutrition can do a lot to protect our brains.

We all lose function in our brains as we age. The role of nutrition and lifestyle is to slow this loss of function. Of all the many nutrients that can help augment the function of our brain and protect it from the ravages of aging, acetyl-L-carnitine is one of the most important.

Many people ask, "When do I need to begin to start taking supplements to protect my brain?" The question again returns to our definition of optimal health: do the cells of your body have the freedom to do what they want? Do they have enough nutrients to protect themselves from the many toxins in our environment? Do they have the optimal ability to protect themselves from daily stresses? The time to begin optimal brain nutrition is in the womb.

A *minimal program for lifetime brain protection would include the following nutrients:*

B complex	50 mg
Vitamin C	1,000 mg
Vitamin E	400 IUs
Magnesium	400 mg
Zinc	25 mg
Selenium	200 mcg
Boron	3 mg

A very important nutrient for brain function is fatty acids. A large percentage of the brain is made up of fats in the form of phospholipids. Bound into these phospholipids are the omega-3 fatty acids from fish, EPA and DHA. While those who consume flaxseed oil may be able to raise their levels of EPA, DHA levels are harder to raise without actually consuming this fatty acid. For those who do not want to consume fish and fish oils, there are now plankton-derived supplements of DHA. However, in my practice, I have found that both EPA and DHA are beneficial.

Fats needed daily for brain function:

1 tablespoon flaxseed oil
300 mg each of EPA and DHA

Supplements can also play an important role in protecting the brain from the damaging effects of stress. To the above recommendations I often add the following nutrients and herbs to help cut down on the likelihood of the body's going into a stress response that will damage the brain. These nutrients not only protect the brain from stress, they make it less likely that you will overreact in the first place. Such overreaction at times becomes a vicious cycle, where a lack of nutrients throws us into a stress response that further damages our neurons.

Advanced brain-protective supplements:

Acetyl-L-carnitine	250–1,000 mg per day
Phosphatidyl serine	200–300 mg per day
GABA	500–1,500 mg
Taurine	1,000 mg or through shellfish (rich in taurine)
Chamomile tea	1–3 cups per day (steep in closed pot to retain therapeutic essential oils)

I also recommend Epsom salt baths as a way to relax the body and help protect it from stress. Epsom salt baths are a great way to give the body nerve-protecting magnesium. For the Epsom salt baths, buy half-gallon containers of Epsom salts. Run a warm bath and put half of the container (1 quart of Epsom salts) into the bath. Put on some relaxing music and stay in the bath for at least fifteen minutes. You will feel your stress hormone levels going down! You will find sleep more restful after an Epsom salt bath. I also have many clients who work at home, and sometimes they break up their stressful day with an Epsom salt bath in the afternoon.

It is also very important for older adults to protect their brains by making sure their blood pressure is under control. High blood pressure shrinks the brain and accelerates brain aging and the loss of brain function.[100]

While nutrients help the brain, use them in the context of this ten-point plan for overall brain wellness. Here it is:

TOP TEN WAYS TO MAXIMIZE BRAIN HEALTH

❶ *Take key brain nutrients.* Optimizing your intake of nutrients that protect the brain is crucial for long-term brain health.

❷ *Manage stress.* Stress is the number one enemy of brain health, for stress hormones destroy brain cells.

❸ *Exercise.* This helps the body protect itself from the deleterious effects of stress and increases circulation to brain.

❹ *Use your brain.* Studies show that those who use their brain regularly—whether doing crossword puzzles, watching Jeopardy, engaging in thought of any kind—are less likely to develop brain degenerative diseases such as Alzheimer's.

❺ *Avoid pesticides in foods.* These compounds have been linked to an increased risk to brain diseases such as Parkinson's disease.

❻ *Limit exposure to toxic chemicals in your environment, at work, and at home.* These are also compounds that damage the brain.

❼ *Don't drink alcohol, which in any amount damages brain tissue.* Also avoid coffee, ephedra, and other stimulants that overstimulate the brain.

❽ *Cultivate a spiritual life,* which is crucial for good mental health and less stress.

❾ *Maximize liver health.* If your liver is doing a good job of getting rid of toxic material that comes from both the environment and our own body's metabolism, these toxins are less likely to damage the brain.

❿ *Avoid medications as much as possible,* both prescription and over the counter. They have side effects that negatively affect the health of the liver and the brain when taken over the long term.

Acetyl-L-Carnitine Slows Brain Aging

Acetyl-L-carnitine is a special form of carnitine that has the particular ability to optimize brain function. Acetyl-L-carnitine is able to cross into the brain more effectively than regular carnitine. It therefore enhances brain-cell function much better than regular carnitine. As we age, acetyl-L-carnitine levels in our brains go down, and for optimal brain function, supplements of acetyl-L-carnitine become mandatory. Particularly for those over forty, acetyl-L-carnitine is the preferred form of carnitine.

The research on acetyl-L-carnitine is nothing short of extraordinary. Although most of it has been done in animals, there are a handful of human studies as well. Acetyl-L-carnitine prevents the deterioration of the brain during stress, and it helps the aging brain function better. Acetyl-L-carnitine also helps prevent damage that can occur to nerve cells when there is a lack of oxygen in the brain. It is therefore of no surprise that acetyl-L-carnitine is very helpful for stroke victims, who have been found to recover better on 1,500 mg of acetyl-L-carnitine per day.[101]

Acetyl-L-carnitine acts in many ways to prevent the deterioration of brain cells that normally happens with age. It acts as a powerful antioxidant, increases levels of a very important messenger molecule called acetylcholine, and provides the brain with healing energy. As we have seen with carnitine, giving cells energy is a wonderful thing. When a cell has enough energy, it can do what it wants and develop itself to the fullest. When a cell lacks energy, it dies. This is particularly bad when it comes to brain cells, because when they die, they are nearly impossible to replace.

The best thing about acetyl-L-carnitine is that it is completely natural. Because of this, it is completely nontoxic. And acetyl-L-carnitine, like all natural compounds, works through many pathways to help keep the body well. When the body weakens, it does so at many points, not just in one particular area. That is why acetyl-L-carnitine and the natural medicine of which it is a part is so superior for disease prevention. No drug will ever work as well as the multitalented acetyl-L-carnitine at slowing brain aging or promoting brain health, because no drug can match its breadth of influence on brain function.

Acetyl-L-carnitine protects against the loss of receptors on brain cells that normally occurs with aging. These receptors on brain cells allow the neurons in the brain to talk to each other. The better our brain cells can talk to each other, the better the brain works. It is like having a broken phone in your house—you don't know if someone is calling you or not. So it is with the receptors on nerve cells—if they are broken, nerve cells can't hear signals and the brain does not work as well. Acetyl-L-carnitine is like the phone guy who makes sure the phones themselves are working. Acetyl-L-carnitine also works on the wiring—the way that brain cells send their signals to each other.

Neurotransmitters are the signals sent between nerve cells, also known as neurons. Neurotransmitters are chemicals. Within a nerve cell or neuron, information is sent with an electrical charge. When the message travels between nerve cells, however, it is translated into a chemical—a neurotransmitter—that is sent from one neuron to the next. The subtle interactions between the electrical and the chemical methods of transmitting messages in our 50 billion neurons allows for the fine gradations of function that makes a ballet dancer more graceful than a robot, and the human brain infinitely more creative than a computer.

These signals sent between the neurons are like smoke signals. First, you have to be able to make the fire that can make the smoke. Then you have to be able to control the smoke into a signal. Then, you have to hope that you are sending the signal to someone who understands this form of communication. Acetyl-L-carnitine helps all these equivalent activities in neurons happen effectively.

So, acetyl-L-carnitine does three really remarkable things for your brain and all of your nervous system, including:

➤ Keep neurons healthy and energetic

➤ Help neurons send and receive signals

➤ Protect neurons and their receptors from the damage inflicted by stress

Simply put, acetyl-L-carnitine does everything a nutrient could do to keep your brain functioning optimally.

Because the nerve cells in the brain regulate stress and the aging process, keeping them optimally healthy will slow the aging process as well. So acetyl-L-carnitine not only protects the brain, but the entire body as well.

MORE WAYS ACETYL-L-CARNITINE PROTECTS THE BRAIN

Acetyl-L-carnitine significantly reduces the amounts of damaged fats such as lipofuscin in the brains of aged rats. This is a key sign that it is slowing the aging process in the brain. As lipofuscin builds up in the body, the body ages.[102]

According to animal studies, acetyl-L-carnitine maintains our ability to learn and interact positively with others as we age. In other words, it allows us to teach old dogs new tricks and make them happier throughout the process.[103] It probably does this through its overall beneficial effects on brain function.

Acetyl-L-carnitine increases levels of nerve growth factor (NGF)—an important brain-healing compound. Acetyl-L-carnitine also increases the ability of the body to use NGF more effectively. NGF plays a key role in preserving neurons, especially those that make the valuable brain messenger chemical acetylcholine. Acetyl-L-carnitine also helps neurons in the hippocampus respond better to NGF. As we age, we respond less effectively to NGF, and acetyl-L-carnitine reverses this decline.[104]

Acetyl-L-carnitine also helps maintain the myelin sheath around the nerves that is important for their health and function. This is important, because without myelin, our nerves cannot transmit their messages at optimal speed. This suggests that acetyl-L-carnitine might be useful in the treatment and prevention of multiple sclerosis. More studies are needed here.

Another thing acetyl-L-carnitine does is preserve the genetic information (DNA and RNA) in our cells, especially that found in the mitochondria. DNA and RNA are very important for the longevity of these energy centers and for keeping them running well and supplying our cells with energy. Acetyl-L-carnitine, in both the heart and brain, appears to protect this genetic information that is so important for health and longevity.[105]

Acetyl-L-carnitine helps brain cells use alternative energy sources, such as lipids or ketone bodies. The brain prefers glucose as its main fuel. Taking acetyl-L-carnitine helps our brain cells adapt to lower levels of glucose in the blood, which can sometimes occur between meals or during hypoglycemia. By so doing, it helps the brain maintain a constant supply of energy needed for optimal health and longevity.[106]

COMMON QUESTIONS ABOUT ACETYL-L-CARNITINE

When should someone start taking acetyl-L-carnitine?

As early in adulthood as possible. College age is a good time. While I believe it is an essential supplement for everyone over forty who wants optimal brain health and longevity, the damage to the brain from stress begins earlier, in the college years for many. So for those who can afford it, I recommend taking acetyl-L-carnitine during stressful times (studying, exam times) throughout one's twenties and thirties, and regularly after age forty. Brain aging starts young. If we are going to slow it down, we have to start optimizing nutrition and lifestyle as soon as possible. Only then can we get the best handle on preventing the loss of brain function later in life.

How much does acetyl-L-carnitine cost?

Acetyl-L-carnitine is somewhat expensive, and I hope to see prices come down soon so that it will become more affordable to the many who can benefit from it. This may be the main limiting factor for many who want to take it. When you compare the cost of a dose of acetyl-L-carnitine (500 mg) to the price of a cup of coffee, however, you realize that it costs less, energizes the brain in a much more beneficial way, and has none of the downside of coffee. A lifetime of taking acetyl-L-carnitine will leave you with a much healthier brain and body than a lifetime of drinking coffee, so make the switch if possible.

Is there anyone who should not take acetyl-L-carnitine?

I do not recommend that acetyl-L-carnitine be taken without supervision in someone with epilepsy or someone who is manic-depressive (bipolar). Such people do not always need more energy in their brain cells.

Are there any side effects to taking acetyl-L-carnitine?

One of the side effects of taking acetyl-L-carnitine regularly is more vivid dreams at night. Some enjoy this while others do not. Adjust your dose of acetyl-L-carnitine to correspond with how much you like to dream!

Top Ten Brain Nutrients

Acetyl-L-carnitine is my favorite brain nutrient, but I do not want you to think that it is the only nutrient you need for maximal brain health. There are many others that we need for optimal brain health, and acetyl-L-carnitine works best when it joins forces with these other nutritional brain boosters.

Here are my top ten favorite brain nutrients:

❶ *Acetyl-L-carnitine.* The most important nutrient for maintaining optimal brain health. Recommended intake: 250–1,000 mg per day.

❷ *Phosphatidyl serine.* The crucial partner with acetyl-L-carnitine for optimal brain health. Recommended intake: 100–300 mg per day.

❸ *EPA and DHA.* These crucial fatty acids are needed for so many different brain cell functions. DHA is probably the most important of all to get, as the body has the greatest difficulty making this fatty acid. Recommended intake: 500–1,000 mg of EPA and DHA combined per day.

❹ *Magnesium* is critical for the health of the brain. Recommended intake: 400 mg per day.

❺ *Folic acid and B_{12}.* I know, these are really two nutrients, but they work together in such an interwoven pattern that you should always think of and take them together. Many cases of depression and dementia have resolved when optimal doses of these nutrients have been used. Recommended intake: 400–2,000 mcg per day of each.

❻ *Zinc.* Brain function depends to a great degree on having enough of this critical mineral around. Recommended intake: 25 mg per day balanced with 2 mg copper sebacate per day.

❼ *Vitamin E.* This remarkable nutrient may be best known for preventing heart disease and keeping immune function strong, but vitamin E has also been shown to help slow the progression of Parkinson's and Alzheimer's disease. Recommended intake: 400 IUs per day.

❽ *Vitamin B$_6$* is crucial for the metabolism of all of the chemicals needed for nerve-cell communications. Recommended intake: 50 mg per day.

❾ *CoQ10.* A wonderful nutrient for keeping nerve cells energized and protected. Recommended intake: 50–100 mg per day.

❿ *Phosphatidyl Choline.* A key liver and brain nutrient that helps overall nerve-cell function. Recommended intake: 500–1,000 mg per day.

TOP TEN BRAIN HERBS

Herbal medicines are some of the most exciting ways to promote brain health and help manage brain ailments. While the nutrients are the most important, the herbs are very useful as well. First give your brain what it needs most—especially acetyl-L-carnitine, phosphatidyl serine, and DHA. Then make sure you have enough of all the other nutrients. When that is done, consider moving on to these herbs. You do not need to take all of these. Try them one at a time to see which one(s) benefit you the most.

❶ *Reishi* is my personal favorite brain herb. This remarkable mushroom has benefits that help balance the entire body and have wonderful balancing effects on brain function.

❷ *Ginkgo* is perhaps the best-studied herb for enhancing circulation to the brain and increasing the health of brain cells.

❸ *Milk thistle* is very important for enhancing liver function, which is crucial for long-term brain health. If your liver is not getting rid of toxins, these will damage your brain over time.

❹ *Rosemary* is powerful antioxidant, wonderful for enhancing mental energy and overall brain health.

❺ *Kava* is a wonderful plant for helping decrease the damaging effects of stress on the body and the brain in particular.

❻ *Gotu kola* (also known as Centella asiatica) is a plant that has stress-managing and alertness-enhancing effects. It may also help the brain make more of the valuable neurotransmitter, acetylcholine.

❼ *Rhodiola rosea* is a plant that has been found to have dramatic effects on enhancing mental function and energy, according to animal studies and my own clinical experience.

❽ *Grape seed extract* is another wonderful plant extract that helps increase circulation to the brain and protect brain cells.

❾ *Bilberry extract* works well to support the health of the delicate capillary network that feeds the brain.

❿ *Valerian* is not to be underestimated as a brain herb. Valerian is great for stress management during the day, and is great for people of high mental energy who want to prevent themselves from burning out.

Stress

Stress accelerates aging. One of the main ways it does this is by weakening important areas of the brain such as the hypothalamus and the hippocampus. The hippocampus is a very important area of the brain where much of our new learning takes place. It is no larger than the nail on your pinky. Damage it, and your short-term memory and learning ability will falter, or in extreme cases, go completely. The reason stress is so damaging to the hippocampus is that stress hormones burn it out. When this happens, it triggers a whole cascade of events that accelerate aging.[107]

Stress is the main enemy of the hippocampus and the brain as a whole. One day while racing to the airport, I looked at my friend who was driving. He was vexed. "Relax," I said. "This is not worth damage to your hippocampus."

He laughed. I explained the whole story. "You're right," he said, "it's not."

So the big question to ask yourself whenever you are under stress is, "Is this worth damage to my hippocampal neurons?" The answer should always be no.

Remember: stress is really your reaction to the situation, not the situation itself. So there are three things to do to preserve brain function:

➤ *Avoid stress as much as possible.*

➤ *Learn to remain calm under potentially stressful situations.*

➤ *Take nutrients that preserve brain function under stress, as outlined above. A diet with protein at each meal and lower in sugars and starches is highly recommended for those under stress. The two most important nutrients to take are acetyl-L-carnitine (250–2,000 mg) and phosphatidyl serine (100–300 mg), but all brain nutrients, including zinc, magnesium, antioxidants, and B vitamins, should also be in good supply. GABA, taurine, kava, and valerian can also be used to protect the brain from stress.*

The following is speculative, but should give you a good idea of what kind of damage stress can do to this most delicate part of your brain:

EVENT	NUMBER OF HIPPOCAMPAL NEURONS LOST
Getting angry about driver who cut you off	3
Getting angry over misplaced keys	5
Having an argument with your spouse	8
Working past the daily capacity of your brain to handle stress	10 per day
Ongoing emotional stress or worry	10 per day

Again, this is speculation, but I feel these numbers are fairly reasonable. The point here is to realize that the way you react each day affects your brain health, and that senility and loss of brain function are things over which our daily behavior has a great deal of influence.

We must become aware of all the stress in our lives and measure our reaction to it. Fish do not know water exists until they are taken outside of it and begin to suffocate. Those under a lot of stress do not know it exists until it begins to kill them. Unfortunately, the way stress kills us is very subtle, and we often do not see it until it is too late.

Remember my analogy used earlier about a plane flying from Los Angeles to New York? If it is off by a few degrees, it ends up in Boston. If throughout our lives we are under stress by just a bit too much, or lack just enough of the nutrients that manage stress, our destination of health at the end of our life will be profoundly different. Memory, immune function, and organ health will all be profoundly weakened.

The most protective compound you can give your brain is energy, which is why the brain-energizing nutrients like acetyl-L-carnitine are so protective. Notice how it takes initiative—energy—to tell a noisy person near you in a theater to be quiet? Brain cells also need energy to send signals to other cells to be quiet when the messages they send become too loud. If neurons don't have the energy to turn off other cells, they can be killed by the stress of too many incoming messages. Acetyl-L-carnitine, by giving neurons energy, allows neurons to stand up for themselves and send out the molecular equivalent of the phrase "shut up." In so doing, acetyl-L-carnitine plays one of its most valuable antiaging roles.

It is the same way in our lives. People are really like individual neurons, especially at their desks. They receive many incoming messages that can annoy them and burn them out.

In my office, I often have a "no phone day." This can be any particular day when I take my phone, turn off the ringer, and put it out of view. This way I cannot hear whether it is ringing or see the flashing light to know there are messages. I love it! It protects me from messages that are distracting and stressing me and allows me to be much more relaxed, focused, and productive.

I think that if businesses had a day when no one talked on the phone, they would be much more productive. I think all of us are addicted to the stress and distraction of the phone. We get used to just working on things in spurts, not in a long, even manner. The phone-based existence of business has dictated that. Do not let the phone rule you—rule it.

We think that stress is a necessary part of getting things done. This is not true. There is a joke about a man who goes into a doctor's office and complains about his uncle. "He thinks he's a chicken." "Bring him in," the doctor says, "I think I can cure him." "I can't," the man says. "We need the eggs."

We view stress the same way. We think that it is okay to put up with it. We are getting so much done! "I may be killing myself, but the company advanced this year." So we lose a few neurons—we have more material goods because of all the pressure we have put on ourselves. We burn out our brains, but our net worth increases. Such thinking is problematic. If we balance our lives better and nourish our brains with optimal levels of nutrients, we can be successful without letting our body be so damaged by stress.

You can be very productive without destroying yourself. Do one thing at a time without distractions. Remain the master of your incoming messages in your neurons with acetyl-L-carnitine to energize you. You will be able to create simpler working strategies that will get you better results.

A spiritual life is also very important for managing stress and keeping mental energy balanced. Emptiness can gnaw at the soul and fell the most beautiful mind and body. If you don't have answers to life's most basic questions, start there first, because that is the place where health starts.

Healthy relationships are also crucial to stress management. Emotional stress will undermine you regardless of how successful the rest of your life is. Work all of these things out with a therapist or your spiritual advisor.

Stress at a certain level is needed. We need some activity to promote brain-cell interaction. Learning, memorizing, even memorizing the license plate of someone in front of you just to see if you can remember it in an hour—these are useful games to play to stimulate mental strength. If you don't use your brain, you will lose it.

Too much stress is destructive. Be independent of the weather, the traffic, and the mistakes of others. Don't let such things rule your mood. You will live longer and have a better-functioning brain and healthier body.

A few years ago, I was in the office of the remarkable physician Dr. Emanuel Revici, who was then ninety-eight. I was taping an interview with him, and dropped my heavy recording equipment on his beautiful large desk. It made a sizeable dent. Dr. Revici said, "Don't worry about it." That's why Dr. Revici has now lived past one hundred with a sharp mind. He doesn't worry about it.

Carnitine and Acetyl-L-Carnitine in Natural Medicine

In this section, we will look at the many health problems that carnitine and an overall program of optimal nutrition can help treat. We will start by looking at the heart, and then examine all the other health problems where carnitine can play a healing role. Let's begin by looking at a healing strategy that underlies my overall approach to generating wellness: energy therapy.

Energy Therapy

Energy therapy is the most important healing strategy in natural medicine. Energy heals. When the cells of the body have more natural energy, they are able to overcome many ailments, both chronic and acute. As we look at many health problems in the section ahead, understand that energy therapy is always the underlying approach.

Energy therapy is especially effective in people with chronic diseases who have not been helped by medicine, traditional or otherwise. They often have every ailment you can name, and nothing seems to help. Or, they may have no real diagnosis though they may be tired, have a sluggish metabolism, or have a wide range of minor health complaints. When illness gets complex, get simple. Use energy therapy.

Energy is crucial to the health of the body. It is no wonder that nearly every great medical tradition in the world is built upon the nurturing of natural energy—vitality. This is something unrelated to stimulant energy, which can destroy the body in the long run. This is natural, renewable energy that comes from building the body up with supportive nutrients and herbs. Remember: If our body is tired, we can rest and sleep, but if an individual cell runs out of energy, it dies. Accelerated cell death from cells running out of energy is what causes disease and premature aging.

Energy therapy is a humble way of healing. It gives the body more energy and allows the body to decide how and where to use it to build health. Your body wants to be radiantly healthy; if you give the cells of the body enough energy, it can be.

Body cells need energy to:

➤ *Build and repair tissue*
➤ *Take out cellular trash that can poison the body and cause disease*
➤ *Defend the body from bacterial and viral invaders*
➤ *Regulate organ function*
➤ *Help cells talk to each other and create homeostasis*

All of this depends on energy. If there is a lack of energy in cells, these things will not happen, no matter what else you do. The more optimal the amount of natural energy cells have, the more easily all this can happen. It is that simple.

Energy is cellular money. You cannot run a city unless all city workers are paid, and you cannot run a healthy body unless all the cells have abundant energy. Without energy, the cells of the body go on a strike, which we call a disease.

Because energy therapy is a way of letting the body do its own healing, it is supportive, not disruptive, as drug therapy often is. You almost don't need a diagnosis of the chronic disease when using energy therapy. You can call any chronic illness systemic energy deficiency. You will always be right. Energy therapy is not a cure for all these ailments: just a logical starting place. It will do no harm, and it will be anywhere from moderately to remarkably helpful.

Natural medicine is supposed to get to the cause of disease. Energy therapy does that. Whether it is candida overgrowth, chronic fatigue, fibromyalgia, arthritis, or immune weakness, treating the symptoms is not enough. We must try to understand how it all started if we want to have a true solution, and the start of so many diseases is a lack of energy in cells.

Overstressing the body is a main cause of disease, and energy therapy helps to deal with this problem. How? Cells that are particularly susceptible to the damage of stress are neurons, or nerve cells, and much of the disease results because the nervous system in particular is stressed. Stress kills because it does something terrible to the nervous system: it destroys its ability to regulate stress. When the nervous system can no longer regulate stress, stress hormones go too high and destroy the body over time.

Aging is the gradual loss of the body's ability to regulate stress, which results in a loss of health. Increasing energy in cells slows aging by helping the body to regulate stress better, and therefore better maintain health.

Energy stops stress from killing our stress-regulating nerve cells. Energy keeps nerve cells and their receptors better able to stay in control of the body so that stress does not get out of control and cause disease.

Energy therapy is simple: Give the cells of the body an increased ability to make more energy naturally, and let the cells of the body decide what to do. I have tried this in cases of chronic disease when I have run out of ideas, and it has been very helpful. It is not a cure, but I feel that it has helped many people, and it is a logical place to start.

CORE ENERGY THERAPY PROGRAM

Activity

Do moderate exercise that is not too stressful, such as walking. Strength training is also an absolute must. These two forms of exercise should be done as regularly as possible; not to the point of exhaustion but to the point of rejuvenation. For some this will mean ten minutes of exercise three times per week. Others will benefit from more. But some exercise must be done. Exercise is one of the most crucial factors for maintaining the energy-producing ability of cells as we age.[108]

Diet

Protein at each meal, ideally high-quality animal protein from wild game. No sugars, margarine, or refined vegetable oils. Follow the basic principles of the Carnitine Program as outlined above. Consume green-vegetable juices: three six-ounce glasses per day, freshly made from only green vegetables (celery, spinach, dandelion, and zucchini work well). Take MCT oil, one tablespoon with breakfast, and flaxseed oil, one tablespoon with a meal.

Supplements

Carnitine	500–4,000 mg
CoQ10	50–400 mg
Magnesium	400 mg
B complex	100 mg
Vitamin C	2,000 mg
Vitamin E	400 IUs
Selenium	200 mcg

Add these supplements to the above if results are not adequate or symptoms of chronic disease are severe:

Acetyl-L-carnitine	500–2,000 mg
NADH	2.5–10 mg
Creatine	1–5 grams per day
Malic acid	1,000–2,000 mg
Glutamine	4–20 grams

This should be adapted to suit individual needs. Trace minerals such as zinc, copper, and manganese should be given according to results of individual mineral testing.

Now let's look at some more ailments more specifically, and see how energy therapy underlies my treatment for virtually all of these conditions. We'll begin by looking at how carnitine and its companion nutrients promote heart health and treat a range of conditions affecting the heart.

Carnitine and the Heart

The heart pumps blood at the rate of five gallons per minute non-stop, and more when you exercise. To fuel its tireless cells, the heart derives at least two-thirds of its energy from fat. Carnitine, critical for fat burning, is a crucial nutrient for heart health, and a lack of carnitine in the body usually affects the heart first.

Because carnitine is so important at promoting the energy and health of heart cells, it helps prevent and treat virtually every heart condition. Ideally, therefore, anyone interested in optimal heart health throughout their life should keep carnitine levels optimal. We should not wait until we develop heart disease before taking carnitine. We should take it throughout life to keep our hearts in top shape.

Carnitine also raises HDL cholesterol, the protective cholesterol fraction, helping to keep coronary arteries clear. Carnitine lowers high triglycerides and also lowers blood pressure in those with hypertension.

If you have any form of heart disease, you should take carnitine under the guidance of your physician or health care practitioner. This is because carnitine can reduce and even eliminate the need for many heart drugs, and this tapering off of drugs must be done with the guidance of a physician. Ideally, you should work with a nutritionist who can work in tandem with your doctor or with a physician well-versed in optimal nutrition.

Here is a daily supplement strategy that is the bare minimum for everyone who wants optimal heart health throughout life:

Supplements for a healthy heart

Carnitine	500–2,000 mg
CoQ10	50–200 mg
Taurine	1,000–2,000 mg
B complex	50 mg
Vitamin C	1,000 mg
Vitamin E	400 IUs
Magnesium	400 mg
Zinc	25 mg
Selenium	200 mcg
Flaxseed oil	1 tablespoon

Now let's look at specific supplement strategies for a range of heart ailments.

ANGINA

Angina is caused by a lack of circulation in the heart. Carnitine is one of the most important nutrients for treating angina, or any condition that involves suboptimal circulation to the heart.[109] Angina patients respond well to optimized nutrition, and it often reduces their need for many of their medications.

Supplements

Carnitine	1,000–4,000 mg
CoQ10	200–400 mg
Taurine	1,000–3,000 mg
N-acetyl-cysteine	1,000 mg
Magnesium	500–1,000 mg
EPA/DHA	700–1,000 mg
Vitamin C	1,000–3,000 mg
Vitamin E	400–800 IUs
Selenium	200 mcg
Herbs	Hawthorn, cactus, motherwort

CARNITINE CASE HISTORY

Ray, sixty-two, had angina, and was taking nitroglycerin and other drugs for it. Even with the medications, he still had pain in his chest if he walked up a flight of stairs quickly or did simple things like chase his grandchildren around his backyard. With his doctor's approval, I put him on 2,000 mg of carnitine, 300 mg of CoQ10, 400 mg of magnesium, and 400 IUs of vitamin E. I also used the herbs hawthorn, cactus, and motherwort. I also had him add cayenne pepper to his food, which he enjoyed. Cayenne is another heart-helper. Ray also had weight to lose, so I put him on the Carnitine Program Phase I, which helped him lose about a pound per week. After two months on this regime, Ray had more energy, had less pain in his chest, and felt better overall. His physician said that if this improvement continued, he could take Ray off his heart medications. Ray felt more well at each monthly visit he had with me, and was excited about living a long, healthy life and enjoying his retirement to the fullest.

ARRHYTHMIAS

When the heart cannot regulate its rhythm, problems can occur. Nearly one-third of all deaths related to heart disease occur because of arrhythmias. Carnitine is a valuable nutrient for the control of arrhythmias, but the most valuable nutrients are taurine, magnesium, and fish oils, which together have successfully eliminated every case of arrhythmias that I have seen in my practice. Limiting sugars and caffeine and getting adequate protein is also important.

Supplements

Taurine	1,000–3,000 mg
Magnesium	500–1,000 mg
EPA/DHA	1,000 mg
Carnitine	1,000–4,000 mg
CoQ10	200 mg
Vitamin C	1,000 mg
Vitamin E	400 IUs
Selenium	200 mcg

CONGESTIVE HEART FAILURE

Carnitine, especially when combined with CoQ10, is one of the best nutrients for helping treat congestive heart failure. The exercise tolerance of congestive heart failure patients goes up markedly on 900 mg of carnitine per day.[110] In fact, the nutritional management of heart failure with these two nutrients is so effective that it should always be the first therapy of choice—whether medications are used or not.[111] Some have even suggested that physicians who do not use optimal nutrition to treat congestive heart failure be brought up on malpractice charges because they are denying their patients the most effective and proven therapy!

Supplements

Carnitine	2,000–4,000 mg
CoQ10	300–400 mg
Taurine	1,000–4,000 mg
Magnesium	500–1,000 mg
Creatine	1,000–5,000 mg
B$_1$ (thiamine)	200 mg
B complex	100 mg
EPA/DHA	700–1,000 mg
Vitamin C	1,000–3,000 mg
Vitamin E	400–800 IUs
Selenium	400 mcg
Hawthorn extract	3 capsules per day

Carnitine and
Natural Healing

Now that we have seen how carnitine benefits the heart, let's look at how carnitine can play a useful role treating a wide range of other conditions as well.

BRONCHITIS

Whenever there is an infection involving the lungs, I always recommend carnitine as part of the nutritional therapy. Carnitine helps promote lung health, and acts as an antioxidant in the lung.

Supplements

Vitamin A (mycellized liquid best)	50,000 IUs
Vitamin E (mycellized liquid best)	400 IUs
Vitamin C	2,000–5,000 mg
Carnitine	1,000–2,000 mg
Taurine	1,000–2,000 mg
N-acetyl-cysteine	1000 mg
Zinc	25 mg
Selenium	400 mcg

CANCER

Cancer comes in many different forms, and it is best to have a supplement program designed for you by a health-care practitioner who can address your unique needs. But there are certain core nutrients that I feel almost every cancer patient should be taking. I know from hosting a nationally syndicated radio show for many years that so many of you have no one to even suggest a basic regime for supporting health during chemotherapy, radiation, or surgery, so here is a starting list of supplements I recommend to most cancer patients who come to see me.

Supplements

Natural carotenoids (from carrot extract, D. salina algae or other natural source)	50-200,000 IUs
Vitamin A (mycellized liquid)	50,000 IUs weekdays only
Niacinamide	500-2,000 mg
Vitamin C	2,000-10,000 mg and higher
Vitamin E succinate	400 IUs
Carnitine	1,000-4,000 mg
CoQ10	200-400 mg
N-Acetyl cysteine	1,000-2,000 mg
Taurine	1,000-3,000 mg
Magnesium	400 mg
Selenium	400 mcg
Bifidobacteria	1 tablespoon of powder per day with a meal
Herbs	Green tea, astragalus, red clover, dong quai, reishi, burdock root

The form of vitamin C that I use with cancer patients is ascorbic acid, occasionally mixed with magnesium ascorbate to help buffer the acidity for those with sensitive stomachs. I do not recommend the more expensive Ester C form of vitamin C (U.S. patent no. 4,822,816, Inter-Cal Corp., Prescott, Arizona), because it would give too high a dose of calcium at the 10-gram and above dose of vitamin C. Evidence from human studies does not suggest that Ester C offers any advantage over ascorbic acid.[112]

Foods such as garlic, onions, green leafy vegetables, and freshly ground flaxseeds should be eaten regularly by cancer patients. All foods should be organic; that is, grown without the use of pesticides, herbicides, and fungicides. Margarine, fried foods, white-flour foods, sugar, and junk foods should be avoided. Fresh vegetable juices can often be quite helpful but may not be for everyone. Many need to concentrate on more high-quality cooked foods and soups. An all-raw-food diet is not something I often recommend to cancer patients or anyone.

There is no one diet for cancer patients, nor is there one supplement or herbal regime that works for everyone. Each person with cancer is different and requires a unique dietary and supplemental approach. The benefits will vary from an increase in life quality to an increase in life length. These nutrients will do no harm, and these basic guidelines are a good place to start. Be sure to do all of this with the approval and supervision of your health care practitioner.

CANDIDIASIS

The overgrowth of candida albicans is a widespread problem, one that affects both men and women. Carnitine does not kill yeast, nor does it affect the growth of beneficial bacteria in the gastrointestinal tract. What it does do is increase overall energy and promote liver health, both of which are very important in the management of yeast overgrowth.

There are two phases in the management of candida overgrowth: the initial killing phase, when your goal is to quickly reduce the amount of yeast overgrowing in the digestive tract; and the long-term phase, when you are trying to increase overall health so that candida overgrowth will not return.

Candida management requires an entire lifestyle assessment. Exercise is important, as is decreasing stress and getting enough sleep. I know many people who only get an overgrowth of yeast in their system only when they start missing sleep!

The diet that works for candida is the Carnitine Program, modeled of course on the Paleolithic diet—low in carbohydrates, higher in protein, and adequate in essential fatty acids.

INITIAL KILLING PHASE (FIRST WEEK OR TWO)

Supplements

Essential oil of oregano	1–2 drops dissolved in 8 ounces of water taken three times per day
Molybdenum	250-500 mcg
Freshly ground flaxseeds	1–3 tablespoons per day in food or with water
MCT oil	1–2 teaspoons per day with breakfast and lunch
Glutamine	5–10 grams per day
B$_6$	50 mg
Zinc	25 mg
Selenium	200 mcg

Symptoms may get worse as the yeast die off in the initial killing phase. This will usually pass after a week or two. Ideally, one should do all of this with the supervision of a health care practitioner so symptoms can be monitored and appropriate supplement changes made as the yeast die off.

LONG-TERM TREATMENT

Stop the oil of oregano after one or two weeks and add:

Supplements

Beneficial bacteria	Take a high-quality preparation three times per day that is high in acidophilus and bifidobacteria. For severe cases, high doses are needed: 1–3 teaspoons per day of both acidophilus and bifidobacteria preparations. Supplements of bulgaricus can also be helpful.
Vitamin C	1,000 mg
Vitamin E	400 IUs
Carnitine	500–2,000 mg

| Acetyl-L-carnitine | 250–500 mg |
| Phosphatidyl choline | 1,000 mg |

After a month or two, stop glutamine and take beneficial bacteria supplements twice per week. Continue with carnitine, acetyl-L-carnitine, and phosphatidyl choline as long as your budget allows.

The most important supplement for the treatment of yeast overgrowth is the beneficial bacteria. These are crucial for the building up of digestive-tract health. Too much emphasis in treating candida is put on the killing phase alone. The rebuilding phase is actually more crucial, for if you do not build a healthy environment in the gastrointestinal tract, the yeast will overgrow as soon as you stop using the oil of oregano or whatever else your killing agent of choice is.

If you only have two long-term strategies that you can focus upon when treating yeast overgrowth, make it these two: eating a low-carbohydrate diet devoid of sugars, fruit, and fruit juice; and very generously supplement with beneficial bacteria supplements, preferably in the powder form.

CELLULITE

I have seen this condition be helped by carnitine, especially when it is combined with exercise and other nutrients that support fat metabolism. Following the Carnitine Program and losing weight is also important. Results will vary, but it is worth a try.

Supplements

Carnitine	1,000–2,000 mg
Phosphatidyl choline	1,000 mg
Vitamin C	1,000 mg
B complex	50 mg
Vitamin E	400 IUs
CoQ10	50 mg
Flaxseed oil	1 tablespoon
Zinc	25 mg
Gotu kola	1–3 caps of standardized extract or 1–2 droppers of tincture

CHOLESTEROL HEALTH

Cholesterol is a dynamic molecule in the body. It is used by the body for many good things. If this weren't true, why would the body make it? The key, though, is to give the body the right foods and nutrients to keep cholesterol doing only good things.

Most people are worried about how much cholesterol they eat, but this does not matter, as long as they eat it in fresh foods like fresh meats and eggs. Foods liked aged meats, sausages, and ghee can have oxidized cholesterol, which should not be consumed. Keep your foods fresh and use antioxidants like vitamins C and E and you will be fine.

Many also worry about how high their total cholesterol is. More important is the ratio of HDL to total cholesterol, which ideally should be four or lower. HDL cholesterol is protective against the laying down of plaque in arteries throughout the body.[113] Total cholesterol is not as important as the ratio of the HDL to LDL cholesterol, as long as total cholesterol is under three hundred. If your cholesterol is over three hundred, then it can be considered high. The nutritional strategies listed below will help to encourage both a good cholesterol ratio and an ideal total cholesterol value.

The two most critical things about cholesterol health are:

➤ *You want your LDL cholesterol well-protected by vitamins C, E, CoQ10, carotenoids, and other nutrients that keep it beneficial to the body.*

➤ *You want more HDL cholesterol and less LDL cholesterol. The HDL-to-total-cholesterol ratio should be four or less. Three is excellent. Make sure your doctor orders a blood test that will show you this ratio.*

Nutrients and foods that help keep cholesterol protected and beneficial to the body include vegetables of all kinds, green tea, freshly ground flaxmeal and flaxseed oil, garlic, onions, and most herbs and spices.

Supplements that keep cholesterol from damaging arteries

CoQ10	50–100 mg
Mixed carotenoids	50–200,000 IUs
Lycopene	10 mg
Vitamin C	2,000 mg
Vitamin E	400 IUs
Tocotrienols	100 mg
Zinc	25 mg
Selenium	200 mcg
N-acetyl-cysteine	500 mg

Ways to raise HDL and get a good cholesterol ratio include exercising, quitting smoking, and eating more protein and fewer carbohydrates.

Supplements that encourage a good cholesterol ratio

Carnitine[114]	500–2,000 mg per day
Chromium	400 mcg per day
Niacin	100–500 mg (Use the inositol-bound niacin called inositol hexanicotinate in amounts over 100 mg to avoid harmless but annoying flushing.)

CHRONIC FATIGUE

Chronic fatigue is a complex problem. Nutrition alone is not a cure, but it can be very helpful.

There are two salient characteristics of severe, chronic fatigue:

➤ It is not just simple fatigue that goes away when you get a good week of rest.

➤ It does not have one cause but is a complex breakdown of the body's ability to turn food into energy.

Chronic fatigue sufferers usually have a lot going wrong with them: impaired digestion, metabolic difficulty in turning food into energy, and perhaps a viral or heavy-metal load in the body. Often that is just the beginning.

Carnitine is very helpful in treating chronic fatigue. A lack of optimal levels of carnitine—especially in those who are virally or environmentally stressed—may be one of the many causes of chronic fatigue.

An investigation of thirty-five chronic fatigue syndrome (CFS) patients showed that CFS patients have statistically significant lower levels of carnitine. This is important, because carnitine plays many roles in keeping cells energized. Without enough carnitine, a lot can go wrong. Research also shows that the higher the carnitine levels in CFS patients, the less severe their fatigue.[115] As CFS patients' symptoms improve, their carnitine levels go up. The same researchers who found the correlation between low carnitine levels and worsened symptoms in CFS patients gave 3 grams of carnitine per day to thirty chronic fatigue patients. It helped promote increased energy in these patients. The effects of carnitine supplements were completely positive. The longer the carnitine supplements were taken, the more they helped. Twelve out of eighteen parameters studied were improved, and there was no increase in fatigue or negative side effects from taking carnitine, except for one patient who had mild diarrhea.[116] Chronic fatigue patients are also low in acetyl-L-carnitine and benefit from supplementation of this form of carnitine as well.[117]

Children with fatigue caused by neurologic conditions have also been helped remarkably by carnitine. Stopping the carnitine made these children lethargic again, while restarting it made them energetic and alert.[118] These children had normal blood levels of carnitine to begin with, so we now know that a normal blood level of carnitine does not mean that the body has enough.

Fibromyalgia is a condition similar to chronic fatigue. I have seen carnitine prove very helpful in fibromyalgia in doses up to six grams per day. I like carnitine in these conditions because it helps patients to exercise more. I believe that moderate exercise to the point of mild invigoration—not exhaustion—is crucial for the improvement of those with chronic fatigue and fibromyalgia.[119]

I also think that we can begin to think intelligently about preventing chronic fatigue and other conditions that involve fatigue by keeping our cells optimally energized with carnitine and its companion nutrients.

Supplements for Chronic Fatigue/Fibromyalgia:

Carnitine	2–4 grams, preferably as pure carnitine tartrate powder
Acetyl-L-carnitine	500–2,000 mg
Malic acid	1,000–2,000 mg
Lipoic acid	100–300 mg
CoQ10	100–400 mg
Magnesium	400–800 mg
Zinc	25 mg
Selenium	200 mcg
Milk thistle	100–200 mg of standardized extract
EPA/DHA	500–1,000 mg
Bifidobacteria	1–3 tablespoons per day of powder

Magnesium, zinc, and selenium are also important. So are fats such as flaxseed oil and borage oil. Eliminating grains and dairy is often helpful. Herbalist Chanchal Cabrera has taught me the value of black cohosh in fibromyalgia, and I will often recommend a teaspoon per day of a good quality alcohol extract. Cactus is also a useful herb.

Severe cases of chronic fatigue sometimes have such delicate metabolisms that they need to start with much lower doses than the ones outlined above. Sometimes all that some severely afflicted chronic fatigue patients can tolerate is herbal teas. Their bodies cannot handle supplements at first and need to be built up on milk thistle and dandelion root tea. When you do begin, remember that you need to begin with these doses in a balanced way. Take small amounts of carnitine, lipoic acid, and CoQ10 together because they all work together.

Each case of chronic fatigue is unique. Some have parasites, some do not. Some have primarily liver-based problems, while others have more problems with their adrenal glands. Some have all of the above and more. This regime is not a cure-all, but it has been a helpful starting point for everyone I have seen with this debilitating condition.

DEPRESSION

One of the most frequent problems I see as a nutritionist is depression. The results I get vary from the moderate to the remarkable. Mild depression responds best, while severe depression is more difficult to treat but will still see improvement on an aggressive nutritional program.

Acetyl-L-carnitine alleviates depression, according to well-designed studies.[120] I have found it especially useful in depression that is associated with any form of stress. I think that, particularly in the elderly, acetyl-L-carnitine, phosphatidyl serine, folic acid, and B_{12} should be the first choice of treatment for depression.[121]

You may be surprised to see that I do not list St. John's Wort here. I think that there is no question that St. John's Wort works for mild depression. But I am more concerned about giving the brain things that it is made out of first. St. John's Wort affects the brain; phosphatidyl serine *is* the brain—a profound difference. Phosphatidyl serine works much more effectively for depression than St. John's Wort does, and does so by solving a structural problem in depressed brain cells. Take St. John's Wort if you like. It is perfectly safe and helps many improve their mood levels, but it does not get to the core of the problem as effectively as nutrients like phosphatidyl serine, acetyl-L-carnitine, EPA/DHA, folic acid, and B_{12} do.[122] You should try these and all of the nutrients listed below first.

The following are all the helpful nutrients for brain support that I have found useful in treating depression. Start first with the core nutrient program, and then add the additional nutrients one by one if you need them.

Supplements

Core Nutrients:

Phosphatidyl serine	300–500 mg
Acetyl-L-carnitine	500–2,000 mg
EPA/DHA	500–1,000 mg
B complex	50 mg
B_6	50–100 mg per day
Folic acid	1,000 mcg

B$_{12}$	1,000 mcg
Vitamin C	1,000 mg
Vitamin E	400 IUs
Magnesium	500 mg per day
Zinc	15–50 mg per day
Selenium	400 mcg

If the above core nutrients do not offer complete relief, try the following one at a time to see if they help:

| NADH | 2.5-10 mg per day |

NADH is a wonderful nutrient for the brain, but it is expensive. Try 2.5 mg per day to start, and increase by 2.5 mg every week until you reach 10 mg. You should notice an elevated mood and increased memory and mental energy. I am not aware of any reactions of NADH with any medications, but get the okay from your physician first before you take NADH if you are taking antidepressants.

| N-acetyl-tyrosine (NAT) | 300–600 mg |

NAT is much more effective than tyrosine at helping depression. Do not take this with MAO inhibitor drugs or if you have a history of melanoma. This is one of my favorite nutritional supplements for more severe depression.

CARNITINE CASE HISTORY

Gerald came to me with mild but pronounced depression. He was taking antidepressant medications that helped him only somewhat. I put him on 2 grams of carnitine per day and 1,000 mg of acetyl-L-carnitine along with 700 mg of EPA/DHA (fish oils concentrate) and 300 mg of phosphatidyl serine. I also put him on a high-potency multivitamin and convinced him to eat less sugar and no caffeine. I also eliminated wheat products, which I felt were aggravating his depression. He found that he felt so much better that he no longer needed his medication. He threw out his drugs! He felt his overall body wellness increase. His mood swings, which had been severe, were gone. He felt the biggest benefits came from the acetyl-L-carnitine, the phosphatidyl serine, and the change in diet.

DIABETES

Carnitine is a critical nutrient for the management of diabetes. Carnitine levels are lower in diabetics, and their urinary carnitine excretion is increased. Carnitine also helps them counter the deranged fat metabolism that occurs in this disease. Higher levels of carnitine in diabetics are associated with lower levels of glycosylated hemoglobin.[123] An elevated glycosylated hemoglobin is a sign that blood-sugar levels are high and damaging the body, so carnitine obviously helps protect diabetics by keeping glycosylated hemoglobin low. This is a sign that carnitine is promoting optimal blood sugar levels in diabetics. Many studies suggest that carnitine can play many other roles in preventing the complications of diabetes.[124]

Carnitine helps insulin work better[125] and keeps insulin levels lower.[126] These and many other reasons are why carnitine is an essential supplement for those with type II (adult onset) diabetes.[127]

The number one goal for type II diabetics is to eliminate excess body fat, which carnitine helps to do. When a type II diabetic loses weight, insulin metabolism often improves dramatically, and blood sugar–lowering medication is often no longer needed.

While carnitine is thought of primarily as a fat-burning nutrient, carnitine plays a valuable role in promoting optimal carbohydrate metabolism. It is especially important in promoting healthy carbohydrate metabolism in the diabetic heart.[128] Carnitine levels are usually lower in diabetic hearts, and carnitine supplementation appears to prevent the loss of cardiac function that occurs in diabetes.[129] For these and other reasons, carnitine is an essential supplement for diabetics.[130]

Acetyl-L-carnitine is also helpful for diabetics. It is especially useful in the prevention and treatment of the nerve damage (neuropathy) that occurs in up to 50 percent of diabetics.[131] Acetyl-L-carnitine also appears to be able to prevent digestive disturbances that can occur in diabetes as a result of damage to the autonomic nervous system.[132]

The Carnitine Program is also essential for the management of diabetes. Studies of Australian aborigines show that when they return to their native diet high in animal products and low in carbohydrates—especially low in the refined carbohydrates of civilization—their blood sugar and cholesterol levels go down nicely. This native diet gets 64 percent of its calories from animal products.[133]

Supplements

Carnitine	1,000–4,000 mg
Acetyl-L-carnitine	500–1,000 mg
Vitamin C	2,000 mg
Vitamin D	400 IUs
Vitamin E	400 IUs
Chromium picolinate	400–1,000 mcg
Zinc	25 mg
Manganese	5 mg
Copper sebacate	2 mg
Selenium	400 mcg
Taurine	1,000–2,000 mg
Bilberry extract	100 mg
Ginkgo GB 761 extract	120–240 mg

These nutrients often reduce the need for blood sugar–lowering medication. Ideally, such supplementation should only be done by those who monitor their blood sugar regularly and who are taking these nutrients under the supervision of their physician or osteopath.

CARNITINE CASE HISTORY

Rose is a diabetic, age sixty-two, five-foot-five, who came to see me weighing 230 pounds. I put her on the Carnitine Program Phase I: 2,000 mg of carnitine per day and a high-potency multivitamin. In her first week she felt significantly higher levels of energy. She lost an average of two pounds per week in the first three months of her program. She felt that carnitine helped her lose weight much more easily, and saw her weight loss stop whenever she didn't take carnitine. Her blood sugar was also much better controlled while taking carnitine and following the Carnitine Program.

HIGH BLOOD PRESSURE

When blood pressure is high, the combination of carnitine and CoQ10 can be very helpful. For blood pressure–lowering power, however, no nutrient can compare with taurine. Weight loss is crucial for many with hypertension, which is where carnitine plays its most valuable role. Foods such as celery, garlic, onions, and green and yellow vegetables should be eaten liberally. Exercise and weight loss are also important.

The Paleolithic diet is very protective against high blood pressure. Native people groups rarely see a rise in blood pressure throughout their life. This is due to many things, including their low-sodium, high-potassium diets, which are rich in fiber and low in sugar. It also has to do with the fact that meat and all animal protein has a protective effect against high blood pressure.[134] Their increased level of activity is also protective.

Supplements

Taurine	2,000–4,000 mg
CoQ10	50–200 mg
Magnesium	400 mg
Carnitine	500–3,000 mg
B complex	50 mg
Vitamin C	1,000–3,000 mg
Vitamin E	50 IUs
EPA/DHA	500–1,000 mg
Zinc	25 mg
Selenium	400 mcg
Herbs	Hawthorn, reishi, skullcap

HIV INFECTION

Optimal nutrition is an extraordinarily important thing for keeping HIV-positive patients well. I have had a very rewarding practice working with AIDS patients, and they, to a greater degree than any other patient, have a metabolism that demands optimal intake of all nutrients. There are many important things that AIDS patients must do. One of them is to take carnitine and acetyl-L-carnitine.

AIDS patients have low levels of carnitine.[135] This causes lowered energy levels, lowered immune function, and an accelerated loss of immune system cells. Therefore it is critically important that AIDS patients get the carnitine they need if their immune systems are to remain strong. Carnitine supplements have been shown to benefit those with AIDS in as little as fourteen days.[136]

AIDS patients who take the drug AZT (zidovudine) must take carnitine, in doses of 1–3 grams.[137] AZT depletes carnitine, causing a serious shortage in cellular energy. The symptoms of AIDS—muscle weakness, loss of lean tissue, fatigue, and immune deterioration—mimic the symptoms of carnitine depletion.[138]

Giving AIDS patients carnitine has positive results. The most important benefit is that carnitine keeps the immune cells of AIDS patients from self-destructing. N-acetyl-cysteine and nicotinamide (a form of vitamin B_3) work along with carnitine to help protect immune cells from self-destruction in the face of oxidative stress.[139] This is critical for the long-term survival of AIDS patients.[140] AIDS patients given up to 6 grams per day of carnitine experience dramatic increases in immune function. Once again, these benefits of high-dose carnitine supplementation occurred irrespective of what the blood levels of carnitine were. It appears that in serious conditions such as AIDS, there needs to be a much higher level of intake to get adequate carnitine into cells, allowing them to function adequately in the face of this disease.[141] Carnitine may also help the body fight cytomegalovirus infection, which often accompanies HIV infection.

AIDS patients should also take acetyl-L-carnitine, for it enhances immune function through a different mechanism than L-carnitine. It helps promote the health of the nervous system, which in turn helps the immune system function better. AIDS patients given 1,500 mg per day of acetyl-L-carnitine experienced an increase in immune function and a decrease in anxiety, depression, and hostility.[142]

Supplements

Carnitine	1,000–5,000 mg
Acetyl-L-carnitine	500–1,500 mg
Lipoic acid	100–600 mg
CoQ10	50–200 mg
N-acetyl-cysteine	1,200–2,400 mg
Taurine	1,000–4,000 mg
Glutamine	1–10 grams
Natural mixed carotenoids	50,000 IUs

Vitamin C	1–20 grams (very individual)
Magnesium	600 mg
Zinc	15–50 mg
Copper sebacate	2 mg
Selenium	400–600 mcg

Note that the dose for selenium is a bit high, but this is needed in HIV. I have many AIDS patients who have been taking 600 mcg for years with no problems—and have excellent health. The toxicity of selenium is greatly exaggerated, and with HIV you cannot play around—you need the higher dose. Doses over 400 mcg per day should ideally be taken under the supervision of a health care practitioner.

I also use many herbs with HIV patients, but this is a very individual matter, according to their needs. I use astragalus, avena sativa, licorice, milk thistle, and eleutherococcus senticosus most often, usually in the form of alcohol tinctures.

HYPOGLYCEMIA

Hypoglycemia (low blood sugar) is another condition where carnitine is a must supplement. One of the problems that people with poorly regulated blood sugar experience is swings in energy. This often leads to the depression, fatigue, and carbohydrate cravings they experience. Carnitine helps even out energy levels, and one of the ways it does this is by helping the liver burn fat and produce sugar. A study of medical students who were put on a two-day fast showed that carnitine kept blood-sugar levels normal, while those fasting students who did not receive carnitine had blood-sugar levels associated with hypoglycemia.[143] Research also suggests that hypoglycemia can be caused by carnitine deficiency.[144]

Healthy blood-sugar levels are important for more than energy, because recurrent bouts of low blood sugar throughout life can lead to poor brain function later in life. Therefore, it is important not just for energy but for brain longevity that we keep our blood sugar within a normal range.[145]

Those with hypoglycemia should take at least 1,000 mg of carnitine every morning. This combined with the Carnitine Program will virtually eliminate the symptoms of hypoglycemia.

Carnitine	1,000–4,000 mg
Acetyl-L-carnitine	500–2,000 mg
CoQ10	50 mg
Magnesium	400–600 mg
Zinc	25 mg
Chromium picolinate	200–600 mcg
EPA/DHA	500–1,000 mg
Siberian ginseng extract	100 mg
High-quality adrenal glandular	300–900 mg
Herbs	Licorice, schizandra, eleutherococcus senticosus, avena sativa, motherwort

HYPOTHYROIDISM

The thyroid gland makes hormones that help us burn food, stay energetic, and maintain health in many ways. Research suggests that more than 10 percent of the population has undiagnosed thyroid problems.[146] When thyroid hormone output is low, one is said to have low thyroid function or to be hypothyroid. Orthodox physicians often rely entirely on blood tests to determine thyroid function. More progressive practitioners also look at signs of hypothyroidism that include a morning underarm temperature under 97 degrees, constipation, depression, weight gain, and low energy.

Hypothyroidism is one of the most important areas for carnitine supplementation. Those with decreased thyroid function have low levels of carnitine.[147] Lowered levels of thyroid hormone also leads to increased carnitine loss.[148] There is a lot of evidence suggesting that those with low thyroid function can benefit from carnitine supplements.[149] Hypothyroid patients also have elevated levels of fats in their blood, which carnitine will lower.

I have found carnitine to be a must supplement for low-thyroid patients. It helps them increase their energy, lose weight, cut cravings, lower their triglycerides, and increase mental stamina.

Hypothyroid patients often need both forms of carnitine, and benefit when the dose is divided between before breakfast and early afternoon. This helps them keep energy high throughout the day and avoid the 4:00 P.M. energy crash that usually happens.

Supplements

Carnitine	1,000–4,000 mg
CoQ10	50–100 mg
Thyroid glandular	300–600 mg
Vitamin A	10,000 IUs
B complex	50 mg
Vitamin C	1,000–3,000 mg
Vitamin E	400 IUs
Magnesium	400–600 mg
Zinc	25–50 mg
Copper sebacate	2 mg
Selenium	400 mcg
GLA (from borage oil)	240 mg (from a 1,000 mg borage oil capsule)
EPA/DHA	500 mg

CARNITINE CASE HISTORY

Sarah was forty-three when she came to see me with PMS and what seemed to be low thyroid function as indicated by many symptoms: a morning basal temperature of 96.5°, fatigue, cold hands and feet, constipation, high cholesterol, occasional mild depression, and difficulty losing weight. Her physician wouldn't give her thyroid medication, because he only looked at her thyroid function blood tests.

I put her on the Carnitine Program Phase I alsong with 2,000 mg of carnitine per day, 500 mg of L-tyrosine, 400 mcg of chromium picolinate, 400 mcg of selenium, 500 mg of EPA/DHA, 480 mg GLA, 25 mg of zinc, and a high-potency multivitamin. She felt like a new person: her energy and overall well-being increased, her skin felt much smoother, and she lost one pound per week steadily, which made her very happy. She'd had great difficulty losing weight in the past. Her cholesterol also went down, and her PMS and depression were mostly alleviated.

Make sure to use a high-quality thyroid glandular extract from a reputable company. Glandular supplements vary tremendously in quality, but the high-quality ones whose raw materials come from New Zealand have proven valuable in my practice. Ask your supplement company where they get their raw materials for their glandular products before you use them.

IMMUNE SYSTEM ENHANCEMENT

Carnitine boosts immune function. It does this by making the cells of your immune system more energetic and better able to ward off free radicals. Carnitine also increases the number of immune cells that can protect you.[150]

This extra immune power comes from the increased energy that carnitine delivers—and energy is superb cellular fuel for a strong defense against a range of ailments. When your white blood cells have more energy, they have more power to protect you and remove the pathogens that can make you sick. A more energetic immune system keeps the body cleaner from disease-causing elements, just like a more energetic person tends to keep a cleaner house.

There are many disease states, including cancer, where the body can be breaking down muscle tissue. This can lead to lowered immune status. Carnitine can help reverse that loss of lean tissue, and is a very important nutrient in many ailments by helping the body hold on to valuable muscle tissue.[151]

My experience is that high doses of carnitine—4 grams per day and more—are very useful in the management of viral or bacterial illnesses, conditions where high intakes of vitamin C are known to be helpful. Perhaps one of the ways that vitamin C is helpful in boosting immune function is that it increases carnitine levels. Carnitine and vitamin C make a great immune-assisting combination.

Supplements

Carnitine	1,000–4,000 mg
Acetyl-L-carnitine	500–2,000 mg
CoQ10	50–400 mg
Vitamin A	50,000 IUs (for four weeks, then 10,000 IUs)

B complex	50 mg
Vitamin C	2–20 grams
Vitamin E	400 IUs
Magnesium	400–800 mg
Zinc	25–50 mg
Selenium	400 mcg
Glutamine	4–10 grams
Taurine	1–3 grams
N-acetyl-cysteine	1,200 mg
Grape seed extract	100–300 mg
Herbs	Astragalus, reishi, echinacea, red clover, osha

Doses of vitamin A over 2,000 IUs should not be used by pregnant women.

INFANT NUTRITION

A great shift takes place in the baby's body when it is born: instead of burning glucose (a simple sugar) for energy, with the sugar supplied through the umbilical cord, the baby must now rely on its own fat stores for energy. To now rely on long-chain fatty acids for energy, babies need adequate amounts of the fat forklift, carnitine. Carnitine is critical in order for this "metabolic shift" to happen, and for it to be successful. Carnitine helps the baby make ketones it needs for energy and helps to fuel the growing nerve cells in the baby's brain. Carnitine is also needed for the breakdown of fats that the baby needs to meet overall energy requirements.

The concentration of carnitine in the baby is dependent upon the amount of carnitine in the mother. So, for promoting optimal carnitine levels in the baby, eating carnitine-rich foods like red meat or supplementing with carnitine—especially toward the end of pregnancy—would seem like a good idea. Supplementation may be especially important for vegetarian mothers who do not eat meat or milk.

This carnitine optimization in the mother should continue after birth if she is breastfeeding. Infant levels of carnitine will decline if it is not provided through a formula that contains carnitine, or mother's milk. This is especially true with preterm infants.

The carnitine needs of the baby are great. The liver of the baby is only about 12 percent as able to make carnitine as the adult liver. Even at eighteen months, the ability to make carnitine is only 30 percent of where it should be. For these and other reasons, carnitine is an essential nutrient for babies for at least the first two years of life. This is why you see carnitine added to formulas, especially soy formulas. Cow's milk does contain carnitine (though it can be allergenic for many infants), but soy- and rice-based formulas must have carnitine added.

Breastmilk is the best food for babies. Even when the same amount of carnitine that is present in breastmilk is added to formula, breastmilk leads to higher levels of carnitine in the baby. This is because carnitine appears to be more bioavailable in the mother's milk.

Children Can Also Benefit From Carnitine

Children also benefit from carnitine. While we think of carnitine for helping shed weight, it actually helps children grow and recover from illness as well. Two hundred and fifty-five children aged three to six years were given carnitine in an effort to prevent tuberculosis. For two to five months, 122 children were given 600 mg of carnitine per day, while the other 133 children were given a placebo. The children in the treated group gained more weight than the untreated group. Likewise, a group of malnourished infants and children between the ages of eighteen months and six years were given carnitine, and they experienced an excellent recovery of appetite and growth.[152]

INFERTILITY

One of the most important nutrients for sperm to have enough energy to complete their task is carnitine. Carnitine and acetyl-L-carnitine also help promote fertility by helping defend the body from stress. Stress can upset nervous system function and prevent the body from reproducing. Particularly as we age, acetyl-L-carnitine may have a valuable role to play in promoting maximum fertility.

Sperm need carnitine, but they need a lot of other nutrients, too. For maximizing sperm health and male fertility, I recommend the following supplements to men who may have fertility problems.

Carnitine	1,000–2,000 mg
Acetyl-L-carnitine	500 mg
CoQ10	100 mg
Arginine	3 grams
Folic acid	400 mcg
B$_{12}$	50 mcg
Vitamin C	1,000–5,000 mg
Vitamin E	400 IUs
Magnesium	400 mg
Zinc	25 mg
Selenium	200 mcg
Saw palmetto	160–320 mg of standardized extract per day
Flaxseed oil	1 tablespoon per day

INTERMITTENT CLAUDICATION

Intermittent claudication is a condition marked by poor circulation in the legs. It leads to pain upon simple exercise such as walking up a flight of stairs. Carnitine has been proven to be a valuable nutrient in helping increase the amount of exercise that can be done by those with intermittent claudication.[153] Those intermittent claudication patients whose blood levels of acetyl-L-carnitine increase the most after carnitine supplementation combined with exercise will benefit the most from carnitine therapy.[154] Unfortunately, intermittent claudication patients usually do not have the ability to follow their carnitine levels with expensive blood tests. The more reasonable approach is to take carnitine with the accompanying nutrients for at least one month and see if there are any improvements.

Those with intermittent claudication are usually smokers. Smoking is one of the best ways to damage circulation, and all attempts to stop smoking should be made. If blood pressure is elevated, do not use more than 100 IUs vitamin E without physician supervision, as vitamin E can cause a mild rise in blood pressure in some hypertensives. The rest of the nutrients are safe for hypertensives.

Supplements

Carnitine	1,000–4,000 mg
CoQ10	50–200 mg
Lipoic acid	100 mg
Vitamin C	2,000 mg
Vitamin E	100–400 IUs
Magnesium	400 mg
Zinc	25 mg
Selenium	200 mcg
GLA (from borage oil)	240 mg from one 1,000 mg borage oil capsule
EPA/DHA (from fish oil)	500–1,000 mg
Herbs	Cayenne, ginger, grape seed extract, hawthorn berry

LIVER HEALTH

Because the liver is a major site of carnitine manufacture in the body, those with liver disease or impaired liver function need extra carnitine. Those with cirrhosis are in special need of carnitine.

Carnitine is very liver protective, and has been shown in animal studies to protect the liver from poisons that would otherwise destroy the liver and cause death.[155]

Carnitine is one of my most favorite nutrients for dealing with hepatitis, especially hepatitis C. I have seen many people go into remission (normal liver blood tests) after six to nine months on the protocol outlined below.

Supplements

L-carnitine	1,000–3,000 mg
CoQ10	200–300 mg
Lipoic acid	200–400 mg
Folic acid	2,000 mcg
B$_{12}$	2,000 mcg
Phosphatidyl choline	1,000–2,000 mg

Vitamin C	2,000–5,000 mg
Vitamin E	400–800 IUs
Magnesium	400 mg
Zinc picolinate	25 mg
Selenium	400 mcg
N-acetyl-cysteine	1,000–2,000 mg
Taurine	1,000–2,000 mg
Milk thistle	150 mg of standardized extract
Turmeric	300 mg of standardized extract
Schizandra	100–200 mg of standardized extract
Licorice	3 capsules per day

MEMORY ENHANCEMENT

Acetyl-L-carnitine is one of many key memory nutrients. Acetyl-L-carnitine helps preserve the receptors on the cells in our brain that create memory.[156] Acetyl-L-carnitine helps promote optimal attention and learning ability in older adults who take 2 grams per day.[157] Acetyl-L-carnitine also protects the brain from the damaging effects of stress,[158] which is crucial because too much stress weakens our ability to learn and remember.[159]

Supplements

Acetyl-L-carnitine	1,000–2,000 mg
Phosphatidyl serine	300–500 mg
Vitamin C	1,000 mg
Vitamin E	400 IUs
Magnesium	400 mg
Zinc	25 mg
Boron	10 mg
NADH	2.5–10 mg
EPA and DHA	500–1,000 mg
Ginkgo extract	120–240 mg
Bilberry extract	100 mg
Gotu kola	1 dropper of tincture

MITRAL VALVE PROLAPSE

Mitral valve prolapse (MVP) is a benign condition of the heart where the mitral valve does not close completely. This results in less effective blood pumping by the heart. Strengthening the heart with optimal nutrition helps greatly to reduce the symptoms of low energy and lightheadedness that can sometimes occur in those with MVP. It is also very important to eat along the lines of the Carnitine Program, for many of those with mitral valve prolapse often are hypoglycemic. They need to eat more protein and less carbohydrates, and to avoid sugars, caffeine, and other stimulants.

Supplements

Carnitine	1,000–3,000 mg
CoQ10	50–300 mg
Creatine	1,000–3,000 mg
Magnesium	500–700 mg in divided doses
Taurine	1–3 grams
Vitamin C	1,000 mg
Vitamin E	400 IUs
EPA/DHA	500–1,000 mg

There are many valuable heart herbs that can also be used to support the hearts of those with mitral valve prolapse. The most valuable of these are cactus, hawthorn, and an underrated heart herb, motherwort. I often use all three in a tincture my MVP clients take a teaspoon of once per day.

MUSCLE TENSION

Carnitine helps muscles relax. This is probably because carnitine helps give muscles the energy they need to relax. Other ways to help relieve muscle tension is to rub magnesium chloride liquid directly onto tense muscles. This is great for helping acute muscle cramps. Epsom salt baths are also very helpful for prevention and treatment of painful muscle cramps, as is regular exercise.

Supplements

Carnitine	1,000–3,000 grams
CoQ10	100 mg
Magnesium	500–750 mg
Potassium	from food: greens, beans, nuts, seeds
Vitamin E	400 IU from natural d-alpha tocopherol
Kava	1 dropper per day of extract or 100 mg of standardized kavalactones

NERVE DAMAGE AND NEUROPATHY

Some of the most rewarding and moving experiences I have had as a nutritionist is working with people who have had brain damage from strokes, recreational drug use, and car accidents. While recovery is usually not complete, the advantages of using optimal nutrition in healing the damaged brain are remarkable. Both research and my clinical experience suggest that one of the most valuable nutrients to help heal the physically damaged nerves is acetyl-L-carnitine.[160] Animal studies have shown that acetyl-L-carnitine can greatly improve the body's ability to recover and repair nerves after physical trauma.[161] Acetyl-L-carnitine is a very exciting nutrient for application in any kind of nerve damage because it is a real "Renaissance nutrient" when it comes to healing nerves. The many roles acetyl-L-carnitine plays in promoting nerve healing include:

➤ *Promoting the growth and health of nerve cells in many ways*
➤ *Accelerating the maturation of nerve cells*
➤ *Protecting nerve cells from free radicals*
➤ *Activating nerve growth factor, an important nerve cell healing compound made by the body*
➤ *Speeding the healing of damaged nerves in peripheral neuropathies[162]*

Physical Trauma to the Brain

A woman we'll call Kim came to see me a year after her car accident. She had been rear-ended, and her head had severely jerked forward and then back. A year after the accident, she could not remember more than two states out of the union, though she studied a map of the United States often. She spoke slowly and haltingly. She was taking a few supplements and wanted to know if a more aggressive nutritional regime could help—especially since it had already been a year since her accident.

I said maybe, and at worse it would do no harm except to her pocketbook. These brain supplements are expensive! She was taking B complex, some vitamin C, and an antioxidant formula. A nice start. But with brain damage of any kind, you need to get very aggressive with your nutrition.

The sooner you can optimize nutrition for brain injuries, the better. The goal with such optimized nutrition is two-fold: you want to help stop any further damage to the brain that may be progressing since the accident, and you want to help encourage the brain to heal. While some nerve cells are lost and may not be repairable, others may be encouraged to function better and pick up the slack. Making the brain cells you have work better can make an enormous difference. Optimizing nutrition for the brain also helps neurons set up new networks that can bypass damaged areas.

You also want to protect the brain from further damage that can stem from an accident. One study showed that nearly a third of those with Alzheimer's had had a head injury.[163] Head injuries can set off a cascade of events that optimal nutrition can prevent. Wearing bike helmets and head gear during all sports is important for all of us as well.

What was remarkable was that Kim responded well to the regime, even though she began it a full year after the accident, when one might think nutrition would no longer have a therapeutic effect. Here is what I put her on:

Acetyl-L-carnitine	1,000–2,000 mg
Phosphatidyl serine	500 mg
NADH	5 mg
CoQ10	100 mg

N-acetyl-cysteine	1,200 mg
Vitamin C	2,000–5,000 mg
Vitamin E	1,000 IUs
Tocotrienols	100 mg
Magnesium	400 mg
Zinc	15 mg
Selenium	400 mcg
Lipoic acid	100–200 mg
Octacosanol	20 mg
Milk thistle extract	150 mg
Grape seed extract	100 mg
Ginkgo biloba extract	240 mg

This is quite a list, and it is an expensive regime. But I helped her get her supplements at a reasonable price, and she was able to afford it. After six months, she was talking more clearly, and her memory was much improved. After a year, she sounded better still as she talked to me over the phone, telling me of her plans to open her own business. She also told me that when she stopped the supplements for a month, she found that her brain function and memory worsened. This was reversed by returning to the supplements.

So don't underestimate the power of nutrition to heal the brain. There are many stories like this one, and everyone I have dealt with who has had a brain injury has found optimal nutrition to be a positive experience. No one has fully recovered because of nutrition, but all were helped.

Brain cells always want to heal and have maximal function. Just give them an optimal supply of nutrients and give them the ability to do so.

NEURODEGENERATIVE DISEASES: ALZHEIMER'S DISEASE, ALS, AND PARKINSON'S DISEASE

ALZHEIMER'S DISEASE

The research on acetyl-L-carnitine in the treatment of Alzheimer's disease is exciting, but still preliminary. Alzheimer's patients given 3 grams of acetyl-L-carnitine per day for a year show significantly less mental deterioration.[164] Acetyl-L-carnitine slows Alzheimer's progression in thirteen of the fourteen parameters used to measure mental decline in those with this disease.[165] Acetyl-L-carnitine levels in the cerebrospinal fluid increase in Alzheimer's patients who receive it as a supplement, and supplements of it help retard nerve-cell deterioration. Those with Alzheimer's appear to have a decreased ability to make acetyl-L-carnitine, bolstering the evidence that it is a logical supplement for those with this ailment.[166]

There are other nutrients that should be taken as well by the Alzheimer's patient. Phosphatidyl serine is very important, as are lipoic acid, ginkgo extract, vitamin C, and vitamin E.

Avoiding all gluten-containing grains—wheat, oats, barley, and rye—is recommended for all neurologic disorders. Gluten is becoming increasingly suspect as one of the causes of dementia,[167] and it may be a cofactor in the dementia of Alzheimer's disease.

Supplements

Acetyl-L-carnitine	3,000 mg
Phosphatidyl serine	300–500 mg
Lipoic acid	200 mg
Selenium	200 mcg
NADH	10–20 mg
EPA/DHA	500–1,000 mg
N-acetyl-cysteine	1,200 mg
CoQ10	200 mg
B_1 (thiamine)	500 mg
B complex	50 mg
Folic acid	800–1,600 mcg
B_{12}	1,000–5,000 mcg
Inositol	5–10 grams
Vitamin C	1,000–10,000 mg
Vitamin E	800–1,600 IUs
Tocotrienols	100 mg
Bifidobacteria	1 tablespoon 1 or 2 times per day in water or food
Ginkgo extract	240–360 mg of the GBE 761 extract
Bilberry extract	100 mg
Grape seed extract	200 mg
Rosemary	1 teaspoon tincture in water per day

AMYOTROPHIC LATERAL SCLEROSIS (ALS)

I have worked with a handful of ALS patients and have found that nutrition can play a role in slowing the progression of the disease. The medications that are used to treat ALS do not offer much promise, and I have sometimes seen conditions worsen as well as not improve once they are begun. Medications may help the symptoms, but they do not really address the underlying causes of ALS. While nutritional therapy tries to address them, we still have a big problem: we do not really know what causes ALS.

There are a lot of researchers marching up different trails of the ALS story. Some feel the entire problem is autoimmune. Others suspect a virus is at work. Others look to antioxidants and protecting the body from things that overexcite neurons.

ALS, like most health conditions, is actually multifactorial. An aggressive, optimized nutrition program may help slow this usually fatal condition. This therapy is not a cure for ALS. For some it is only mildly beneficial, while others it helps more, but it is harmless and can do only good.

The most important nutrients for those with ALS are antioxidants like vitamin E, lipoic acid, vitamin C, and N-acetyl-cysteine. Also recommended are nutrients that help promote cellular vitality, like acetyl-L-carnitine, NADH, and phosphatidyl serine.

I recommend avoiding all sources of MSG (monosodium glutamate), including soy sauces, hydrolyzed vegetable protein, the meats and snack foods that contain MSG, or the other ingredients that contain it. Organic foods are also very important because pesticides on foods are toxic to our nerve cells. Managing stress, meditation and prayer, and positive visualization are all also important. Believing you can heal an ailment is crucial to your success.

Supplements

Acetyl-L-carnitine	3,000 mg
Phosphatidyl serine	300–500 mg
Lipoic acid	400–600 mg
NADH	10–20 mg
EPA/DHA	500–1,000 mg
N-acetyl-cysteine	1,000 mg

GABA	500–2,000 mg
Magnesium	400 mg
Selenium	400 mcg
CoQ10	200 mg
B complex	50 mg
Vitamin C	1,000–5,000 mg
Vitamin E	800 IUs
Tocotrienols	100 mg
Bifidobacteria	1 tablespoon 1 to 2 times per day in water or food
Octacosanol	10–25 mg
Ginkgo extract	240–360 mg
Bilberry extract	100 mg
Grape seed extract	200 mg
Valerian	10 drops per day of 1:1 alcohol tincture in glass of water

PARKINSON'S DISEASE

There is evidence that nutrition can play a role in slowing the progression of Parkinson's disease. Acetyl-L-carnitine may be one of the key players in the nutritional arsenal, according to animal studies.[168] Acetyl-L-carnitine appears to help the brain release more dopamine and helps nerve cells respond to it more effectively. Acetyl-L-carnitine can have a positive effect on age-related changes in the dopaminergic system.[169]

For the nutritional management of Parkinson's, acetyl-L-carnitine is just the beginning. NADH, a special form of the B vitamin niacinamide, is also very important. The supplement strategy outlined below will not cure Parkinson's, but in my experience it has helped slow its progression. Such aggressive nutritional therapy should be supervised by a health care practitioner.

Supplements

NADH	10–20 mg
Phosphatidyl serine	300–500 mg
Acetyl-L-carnitine	1,000–2,000 mg
Vitamin E	1,000–2,000 IUs

Tocotrienols	100 mg
Vitamin C	2,000–5,000 mg
Zinc	15 mg
Selenium	400 mcg
Lipoic Acid	200–600 mg
EPA/DHA	500–1,000 mg
N-Acetyl-Cysteine	500–1,000 mg
CoQ10	300 mg
Bifidobacteria	1 tablespoon 1–2 times per day in or with water
Ginkgo extract	240–360 mg
Bilberry extract	100 mg
Grape seed extract	200 mg

PMS

I have often seen premenstrual syndrome improve on carnitine therapy. I discovered this when my female clients taking carnitine saw their PMS disappear. Carnitine therapy for PMS works well when combined with other nutrients and herbs. I also use acetyl-L-carnitine for PMS. Research suggests it restores a normal menstrual cycle and promotes female hormonal balance in doses of 2,000 mg per day.[170] Acetyl-L-carnitine probably promotes hormonal balance in women by increasing the health of the hypothalamus in the brain, which in turn regulates the hormonal functions of the body. Acetyl-L-carnitine also promotes the health of the pituitary gland, another important controller of hormonal health.[171]

Supplements

Carnitine	500–2,000 mg
Acetyl-L-carnitine	500–2,000 mg
Phosphatidyl choline	1,000–2,000 mg
Vitamin C	2,000 mg
Vitamin E	400 IUs
N-acetyl-cysteine	500–1,000 mg
Magnesium	400–800 mg
Zinc picolinate	50 mg

B complex	50 mg
B_6	100 mg
GLA (from borage oil)	240–720 mg from 1–3 1,000 mg borage oil capsules
Vitex-Alfalfa Supreme (from Gaia Herbs)	1–3 droppers

REYE'S SYNDROME

This rare but quickly fatal disorder in children may be prevented if children have optimal levels of carnitine and arginine in their body. Children with Reye's syndrome have significantly lower levels of carnitine, and these low levels of carnitine may be one of the causes of the progression of the disease.[172] Carnitine supplements are highly recommended in this condition. Five hundred milligrams two to three times per day is a suggested dose. Better still would be to give carnitine, arginine, and many other nutrients by injection for the best possible management of Reye's. This must be done under the supervision of a nutritionally oriented—or at least nutritionally cooperative—physician.

STROKE

Many Americans are affected by stroke every year, and there is significant evidence that acetyl-L-carnitine can help promote a better recovery. Animal studies suggest that treatment with acetyl-L-carnitine can improve neurologic function after a stroke if supplementation is started immediately.[173]

Supplements

Acetyl-L-carnitine	3,000 mg
Phosphatidyl serine	300–500 mg
NADH	10 mg
Vitamin A	10,000–25,000 IUs
Vitamin C	1,000–3,000 mg
Vitamin E	400–800 IUs

Magnesium	400 mg
Selenium	400 mcg
N-acetyl-cysteine	1,200 mg
Ginkgo biloba extract	240–360 mg
Grape seed extract	100–300 mg
Bilberry extract	100–200 mg

SURGERY

One of the most powerful applications of optimal nutrition is strengthening the body in preparation for surgery, be it major or minor. Optimizing nutrition before surgery minimizes complications, lessens scarring, and speeds healing. The physicians with whom I work are always impressed by how well healing occurs when the body is given optimal doses of all key healing nutrients. While zinc, vitamin A, and vitamin C are the three most important nutrients, all of them are critical for the growth and healing of new tissue.

Carnitine, CoQ10, and other antioxidants are also crucial. They help prevent damage to the heart that can occur during low levels of oxygen, which can occur during surgery. One gram of carnitine per day given to patients in the days leading up to surgery enhanced their hearts' ability to remain healthy throughout the stress of surgery.[174]

Acetyl-L-carnitine is also valuable for protecting the body during surgery.[175] It is a crucial supplement for those undergoing major surgery because it protects the brain from the lack of oxygen that sometimes occurs under total anesthesia. This often occurs during heart bypass surgery. Such lack of oxygen damages brain cells, sometimes leading to irreversible memory loss. Acetyl-L-carnitine helps prevent this.[176]

I do not recommend high doses of vitamin E the week before or two weeks after surgery, even minor surgery. It is my experience that this valuable nutrient is inappropriate in high doses around surgery, as it may in fact slow the healing of some kinds of surgical procedures, and may undesirably thin blood during surgery. Fish oil supplements should also be avoided for the month prior to and following surgery, as they may also thin the blood inappropriately.

The diet before surgery should have quality protein at each meal. This is not the time to fast or experiment with low-protein diets. Protein is perhaps the single most important nutrient to get in optimal amounts before surgery, for it is the nutrient the body needs most to repair tissue. Two to three four-ounce servings of protein per day is adequate for most people before surgery.

More Americans die every year from hospital infections than from car accidents and homicides combined. This could be greatly reduced by the optimal nutritional program outlined below. One third of the elderly have nutrient deficiencies that impair immune function, and even a simple multivitamin can help augment their immune function before surgery. If deadly hospital infections are to be stopped, it is also important for doctors and nurses to wash their hands more regularly than 40 percent of the time.[177]

Supplements

Carnitine	500–2,000 mg
Acetyl-L-carnitine	500 mg
CoQ10	50–100 mg
Phosphatidyl serine	300 mg
Vitamin A	50,000 IUs (liquid mycellized best)
Vitamin C	1,000–5,000 mg
Magnesium	400 mg
Zinc	25–50 mg
Selenium	400 mcg
N-acetyl-cysteine	1,000 mg
Glutamine	3,000–5,000 mg
Arginine	1,000–5,000 mg
Taurine	1,000–3,000 mg
Astragalus	1 dropper of tincture
Gotu kola	1–3 capsules of standardized extract or 1–2 droppers of tincture
Other useful herbs	Avena sativa, motherwort, valerian, kava

TRIGLYCERIDE LOWERING

Triglycerides are a class of fats in the blood that are getting increased attention from cardiologists. Keeping them below 100 is important for heart and artery health. When they are 100 or higher, risk of heart disease doubles.[178] An optimal triglyceride reading is probably somewhere in the neighborhood of 75, although blood tests still say anything under 150 is fine, a figure that I disagree with. A healthy diet, exercise, and carnitine are all excellent at keeping triglycerides in an optimal range.

Eating fewer carbohydrates in particular is a great way to lower your triglycerides. A review of twenty-seven studies shows that diets high in carbohydrates raise triglycerides and lower HDL cholesterol, both changes marking an increased insulin resistance and higher risk for heart disease.[179] One can find studies showing that diets high in carbohydrates—if they are high in fiber as well—may help blood-sugar metabolism.[180] Those studies are the exception, however. Most studies show that a diet high in sugars and starches worsens insulin metabolism and raises triglycerides. So follow the Carnitine Program and eat a low-carbohydrate diet to lower your triglycerides to below 100.

If your triglycerides are very high, say above 500, don't think that you need drugs to lower them. Go on the Carnitine Program Phase II and cut out all fruit and fruit juices. Fruit is particularly troublesome for those who are likely to have high triglycerides.

Supplements

Carnitine	1,000–4,000 mg
EPA/DHA	700–1,000 mg
Niacin	400 mg (use the inositol hexanicotinate form in amounts over 100 mg to avoid the harmless but annoying flushing reaction)
Pantethine	600–900 mg
Vitamin C	2,000 mg
Vitamin E	400 IUs
Chromium	400 mcg
Gugulipid	100–200 mg

Trace minerals such as zinc and copper are also helpful and should be tailored to individual needs. Diet and exercise should not be forgotten with all of this supplementation. Supplements are helpful, but do not rely on them alone.

All of these supplements are not always needed to get triglycerides below 100. A low-carbohydrate diet with healthy fats like flaxseed oil is the most important strategy. For most people, mildly elevated triglycerides can be lowered with a healthier diet and carnitine. Others with triglycerides well above 150 will need the more aggressive supplement regime outlined above.

CARNITINE CASE HISTORY

Harriet came to see me with a very high triglyceride reading of 782. Ideal triglyceride readings hover around 75, which I told her I could help her attain. I put her on the Carnitine Program Phase II and 2,000 mg of carnitine per day. After three months, her triglyceride reading was 82. Her doctor was impressed with her triglyceride lowering results acheived by carnitine; so much so that he began to use this nutritional therapy with all his hypertriglycedemic patients.

VEGETARIANISM

Carnitine is a crucial supplement for strict vegetarians. It is especially important for young children. Putting young people on a strict vegetarian diet increases the likelihood that they will not get enough carnitine, as well as vitamin B_{12}.[181]

Supplements

Carnitine	500–2,000 mg
Vitamin B_{12}	100 mcg
Vitamin D	400 IUs
Zinc	25 mg
Selenium	200 mcg

Protein supplements—in capsules, tablets, or powders—also help increase the energy and well-being of the strict vegetarians I counsel.

WEIGHT LOSS

Besides carnitine, there are other nutrients one can use to help keep the body burning fat at an optimal rate. I have found that garcinia is helpful when combined with carnitine to promote weight loss. Pyruvate is a new nutritional player that is recently touted for weight loss. I have only begun to use it and cannot give you a definite assessment, yet an informal study has shown that combining pyruvate with chromium, carnitine, and garcinia resulted in excellent weight loss.

I do not expect or even recommend that everyone who needs to lose weight take all of these nutrients. Experiment and see which ones help you the most.

Supplements

Carnitine	1,000–4,000 mg
CoQ10	50–200 mg
Vitamin C	1,000–2,000 mg
Vitamin E	400 IUs
Chromium picolinate	400–600 mcg
Garcinia extract	500–2,000 mg
N-acetyl-cysteine	500–1,000 mg
Selenium	200 mcg
Pyruvate	2–5 grams

In between meals to keep blood sugar even and maintain lean tissue, take two to three 1,000 mg capsules or tablets of predigested amino acids (from whey or other high-biological-value protein) with a glass of water.

Useful Therapeutic Foods

Green tea	1-3 cups daily
Flaxseed oil	1-3 tablespoons per day as a replacement for other fats in the diet
Flaxmeal powder or other fiber supplement	1 teaspoon or more 3 times per day before each meal with 8 oz. water

Top Ten Reasons to Take Carnitine and Acetyl-L-Carnitine

This book has focused on carnitine, yet hopefully you have seen carnitine in the broader context of optimal intake of all beneficial nutrients in addition to the lessons of the Paleolithic diet. Carnitine alone will not make you healthy or conquer any disease. Put into the context of an overall optimal nutrition program, however, carnitine is a very powerful player. Here, then, to end our discussion of carnitine are my top ten reasons to consider taking this nutrient in both of its forms:

❶ *Carnitine slows the aging process!* Every cell in your body—whether it is brain cell, immune cell, heart cell—works better when it has optimal energy available to it. By providing optimal energy to cells, carnitine helps cells live longer and is therefore an important nutrient for a long, healthy life.

❷ *Carnitine keeps triglycerides low and raises HDL cholesterol,* thus helping prevent heart disease.

❸ *Carnitine also helps prevent heart disease by enhancing the overall health of the heart and by helping to prevent cardiac arrhythmias,* the cause of one-third of all heart attack deaths.

❹ *Carnitine helps promote weight loss,* especially when combined with a low-carbohydrate diet.

❺ *Carnitine increases energy levels naturally,* without harm to the body, and without causing side effects or burnout like highly concentrated ephedra supplements. This increases the ability of the body to exercise, and helps protect tissues from damage when they lack sufficient oxygen.

❻ *Carnitine enhances sports performance and endurance and reduces the damage to the body that can occur during exercise.*

❼ *Carnitine and acetyl-L-carnitine both enhance immune function.*

❽ *Acetyl-L-carnitine protects nerve cells from stress and deterioration, and may prevent Alzheimer's disease.*

❾ *Acetyl-L-carnitine naturally increases mental energy and helps relieve depression.*

❿ *Carnitine enhances liver function.* Without optimal liver function, optimal health is not possible.

RECOMMENDED READING

The best effect of any book is that it excites the reader to self-activity.

—Thomas Carlyle

Nutrition and Physical Degeneration
Weston Price, D.D.S.
Keats Publishing
> *Nutrition and Physical Degeneration* is one of the most important nutrition books ever written. Dr. Weston Price circled the globe in the early 1930s and made many striking discoveries about the danger of refined foods like white flour and sugar and the benefits of meat and other animal products. It is one of the most complete reviews of what kinds of diets make people healthy.

Nourishing Traditions
Sally Fallon, Mary Enig, Ph.D., and Pat Connolly
> My favorite cookbook. A must purchase. It will help you create healthy, delicious foods from soup to dessert that are simple to prepare. It is the only cookbook I know that is written by nutritionists and a culinary expert. There is a lot of information about the health-promoting properties of foods throughout this remarkable book.

NeanderThin
Ray Audette
Paleolithic Press
> A fun, slim book that gets to the point: eat like a caveman, feel better, and watch many health problems disappear. Ray is one of the few bold enough to embrace the Stone Age diet and show you how to do it. Call 1 (800) 755-7344 to order.

Power Healing
Leo Galland, M.D.
Random House
> The country's top nutrition physician has written a superb guide that maps out a comprehensive approach to healing yourself naturally. Dr. Galland looks at nutrition, environment, and every other area of your life that you need to examine in order to be optimally healthy. Written in a clear and brilliant style, this book is must reading for anyone who cares about his or her health.

Why Zebras Don't Get Ulcers
Robert Sapolsky, Ph.D.
W. H. Freeman and Company
> A wonderful, fun book on the effects of stress on health. Written in an entertaining style by the brilliant Dr. Sapolsky, it will show you that if you manage stress better, you just might live longer.

Confessions of a Medical Heretic
Robert Mendelsohn, M.D.
Contemporary Books
> This book has sold over 300,000 copies, and with good reason: it is the most brilliant, entertaining, and acerbic warning ever written about the dangers of modern medicine.

Nutritional Influences of Illness, 2nd Edition
Melvin Werbach, M.D.
Keats Publishing
> A compendium of research on how nutrition can treat a range of ailments. A must for any health care practitioner or anyone serious about having the most reliable nutrition information at their fingertips.

Robert Crayhon's Nutrition Made Simple
Robert Crayhon, M.S.
M. Evans and Company, Inc.
  The complete guide to the latest findings in optimal nutrition and an excellent companion to *The Carnitine Miracle*.

DESIGNS FOR HEALTH®

If you are looking for a nutritionist in the United States who can help you create a customized eating program according to your individual needs, please feel free to call Designs for Health. Designs for Health is a company I run that educates nutritionists in cutting-edge clinical nutrition. It is not a franchise, but an educational institution and referral service. So please give us a call, and we will be happy to help you find a nutritionally aware practitioner near you.

If you are a health care practitioner and are interested in learning cutting-edge clinical nutrition with myself and nutrition researcher Linda Lizotte, please contact our main Designs for Health office for more information. Our trainings are held in the New York area as well as Boulder, Colorado. They offer comprehensive training in the use of our range of unique therapeutic diets, as well as the use of nutritional supplements, herbs, and the clinical use of diagnostic nutritional tests. We are also putting much of our training on tape and developing a distance-learning program to help educate those who cannot travel to New York or Boulder.

For more information, write or call Designs for Health at:

Designs for Health Institute
1750 30th Street, #319
Boulder, CO 80301

(303) 415-0229
www.dfhi.com

TOTAL HEALTH MAGAZINE

I am associate editor of Total Health magazine, which I believe to be the finest magazine there is for helping you achieve your goal of optimal health. It is published six times yearly. I write articles for each issue on my latest findings in nutrition and answer reader questions as well. We have assembled the finest practitioners and writers to give you health information that you can use to get yourself well. To subscribe, call or write:

> **Total Health Magazine**
> 165 North 100 East, Suite #2
> St. George, UT 84770-9963
>
> 1 (800) 788 7806

GREAT RESOURCES

The Felix Letter is wonderfully informative and fun to read. Clara Felix comes to you six times a year with her review of the goings on in journals, conferences, and her own personal experiences and those of others. You will get cutting-edge information written in a lively style by one of the country's brightest nutritionists. $12 per year. Sample issue $1. **The Felix Letter**, P.O. Box 7094, Berkeley, CA 94707.

The Price-Pottenger Nutrition Journal is a must subscription. It is a quarterly journal that is one of the true voices about the role of diet in health. It's emphasis on the results of what people groups have been eating for thousands of years gives it a unique perspective. Mary Enig, Ph.D. and other luminaries are frequent contributors. **Price-Pottenger Nutrition Foundation**, P.O. Box 2614, La Mesa, CA 91943-2614. (619) 574-7763.

If you didn't make it to the latest nutrition or herbal conference, Tree Farm Communications has taped it for you. **Tree Farm Communications**, 23703 NE Fourth Street, Redmond, WA 98053. Call for a free catalog: (800) 468-0464.

The *Townsend Letter*'s ten yearly issues are three hundred pages of interesting information on all areas of complementary medicine. Transcripts of in-depth interviews I conduct with health researchers often appear here. The *Townsend Letter* is a must for health care practitioners or anyone interested in having their fingers on the pulse of nutritional medicine. **Townsend Letter for Doctors and Patients**, 911 Tyler Street, Port Townsend, WA 98368-6541. www.tldp.com. (360) 385-6021.

The Paleodiet Symposium Archive page on the internet is a fascinating place to visit if you are interested in the latest discussion on what humans have eaten for the past 2.6 million years. Brilliantly conceived and run by Dean Esmay, this discussion group features the best scientists discussing the most important topic in nutrition: the Paleolithic diet. You can read all the archived discussions at: **http://maelstrom.stjohns.edu/archives/paleodiet.html**.

NOTES

[1] Shigenaga MK, Hagen TM, Ames BN. Oxidative damage and mitochondrial decay in aging. *Proceedings of the National Academy Sciences* (USA) 1994; 91(23): 10771-10778.

[2] Leibovitz B, Mueller J. Carnitine. *Journal of Optimal Nutrition* 1993; 2(2): 90-109.

[3] Costell M, O'Connor JE, Grisolia S. Age-dependent decrease of carnitine content in muscle of mice and humans. *Biochem Biophys Res Commun* 1989; 161(3): 1135-1143.

[4] Monti D et al. Apoptosis—programmed cell death: A role in the aging process? *Am J Clin Nutr* 1992; 55(6 Suppl): 1208S-1214S.

[5] Tesco G et al. Protection from oxygen radical damage in human diploid fibroblasts by acetyl-L-carnitine. *Dementia* 1992; 3: 58-60.

[6] Franceschi C et al. Immunological parameters in aging: studies on natural immunomodulatory and immunoprotective substances. *Int J Clin Pharmacol Res* 1990; 10(1-2): 53-57

[7] Ruggiero FM et al. Effect of aging and acetyl-L-carnitine on the lipid composition of rat plasma and erythrocytes. *Biochem Biophys Res Commun* 1990; 170(2): 621-626.

[8] Lysiak W et al. Quantitation of the effect of L-carnitine on the levels of acid-soluble short-chain acyl-CoA and CoASH in rat heart and liver mitochondria. *J Biol Chem* 1988; 263: 1151-1157.

[9] Cohen M. *Health and the Rise of Civilization*, New Haven: Yale University Press, 1989.

[10] Eaton SB, Eaton SB III, Konner MJ. Paleolithic nutrition revisited: A twelve year retrospective on its nature and implications. *European Journal of Clinical Nutrition* 1997; 51: 207-216.

[11] Reinhold JG. Problems in mineral nutrition: A global perspective. In *Trace Minerals in Foods*, ed. KT Smith, Marcel Dekker, New York, 1988.

[12] Bock G et al. Fruit, vegetables, and cancer prevention: A review of the epidemiological evidence. *Nutrition and Cancer* 1992; 18 (2): 1-29.

[13] Reinhold JG et al. Effects of purified phytate and phytate-rich bread upon metabolism of zinc, calcium, phosphorus, and nitrogen in man. *Lancet* 1973; 1: 283-288.

[14] *Newsweek,* July 21, 1997.

[15] Leonard WR et al. Evolutionary perspectives on human nutrition: The influence of brain and body size on diet and metabolism. *Am J Hum Biol* 1994; 6: 77-88.

[16] Mensink RP, Katan MB. Effect of dietary fatty acids on serum lipids and lipoproteins. A meta-analysis of 27 trials. *Arterioscler Thromb* 1992; 12: 911-919.

[17] Ellis FR, Path MS, Montegriffo V. Veganism, clinical findings and investigations. *Am J Clin Nutr* 1970; 32: 249-255.

[18] Blair R, Misir R. Biotin availability from protein supplements and cereal grains for growing broiler chickens. *Int J Vit Nutr Res* 1989; 62: 773-780.

[19] Subtil JC et al. Dementia due to bacterial overgrowth in a patient with Billroth II anastomosis. *Rev Esp Enf Digest* 1996; 88 (6): 431-433.

[20] Heller RF, Heller R. Hyperinsulinemic obesity and carbohydrate addiction: The missing link is the carbohydrate frequency factor. *Medical Hypotheses* 1994; 42: 307-312.

[21] Franceschi S et al. Intake of macronutrients and risk of breast cancer. *Lancet* 1996; 347: 1351-1356.

[22] Franceschi S et al. Food groups and risk of colorectal cancer in Italy. *International Journal of Cancer* 1997; 72: 56-61.

[23] Siguel EN, Lerman RH. Altered fatty acid metabolism in patients with angiographically documented coronary artery disease. *Metabolism* 1994; 43: 982-993.

[24] Kadrabova J et al. Selenium status, plasma zinc, copper, and magnesium in vegetarians. *Biological Trace Element Research* 1995; 50: 13-23.

[25] Clark LC et al. Effects of selenium supplementation for cancer prevention in patients with carcinoma of the skin. A randomized controlled trial. *JAMA* 1996; 276(24):1957-1963.

[26] Sastre J. Aging of the liver: Age-associated mitochondrial damage in intact hepatocytes. *Hepatology* 1996; 24(5): 1199-1205.

[27] Lockwood K et al. Progress on therapy of breast cancer with vitamin Q10 and the regression of metastases. *Biochem Biophys Res Comm* 1995; 212: 172-177.

[28] Clarkson P. Nutritional ergogenic aids: carnitine. *International Journal of Sports Nutrition* 1992; 2: 185-190.

[29] Swart I et al. The effect of L-carnitine supplementation on plasma carnitine levels and various performance parameters of male marathon athletes. *Nutrition Research* 1997; 17: 405-414.

[30] Dal Negro R. Changes in physical performance of untrained volunteers: Effects of L-Carnitine. *Clinical Trials Journal* 1986; 23: 242-248.

[31] Dragan GI et al. Studies concerning chronic and acute effects of L-carnitine in elite athletes. *Physiologie* 1989; 26: 111-129.

[32] Dragan GI, Wagner W, Ploesteanu E. Studies concerning the ergogenic value of protein supply and L-carnitine in elite junior cyclists. *Physiologie* 1988; 25 (3): 129-132.

[33] Lennon DL. Effects of acute moderate-intensity exercise on carnitine metabolism in men and women. *J Appl Physiol* 1983; 55 (2): 489-495.

[34] Arenas J et al. Carnitine in muscle, serum, and urine of nonprofessional athletes: effects of physical exercise, training, and L-carnitine administration. *Muscle Nerve* 1991; 14 (7): 598-604.

[35] Giamberardino MA et al. Effects of prolonged L-carnitine administration on delayed muscle pain and CK release after eccentric effort. *International Journal of Sports Medicine* 1996; 17: 320-324.

[36] O'Conner JE et al. Protective effect of L-carnitine on hyperammonemia. *FEBS Letters* 1984; 166: 331-334.

[37] Siliprandi N. Metabolic changes induced by maximal exercise in human subjects following L-carnitine administration. *Biochim Biophys Acta* 1990; 1034 (1): 17-21.

[38] Vecchiet L. Influence of L-carnitine administration on maximal physical exercise. *Eur J Appl Physiol* 1990; 61 (5-6): 486-490.

[39] Arenas J. Effects of L-carnitine on the pyruvate dehydrogenase complex and carnitine palmitoyl transferase activities in muscle of endurance athletes. *FEBS Letters* 1994; 341 (1): 91-93.

[40] Marconi C . Effects of L-carnitine loading on the aerobic and anaerobic performance of endurance athletes. *Eur J Appl Physiol* 1985; 54 (2): 131-135.

[41] Sass R, Werness P. Acetylcarnitine: on the relationship between structure and function. *Biochem Biophys Res Commun* 1973; 55 (3): 736-742.

[42] McMillin JB et al. Mitochondrial metabolism and substrate competition in the aging Fischer rat heart. *Cardiovascular Research* 1993; 27: 2222-2228

[43] Brass EP, Hiatt WR. Carnitine metabolism during exercise. *Life Sciences* 1994; 54 (19): 1383-1393.

[44] Avogaro P et al. Acute effects of L-carnitine on FFA and beta-OH-butyrate in man. *Pharma Res Com* 1981; 13: 443.

[45] Huertas R et al. Respiratory chain enzymes in muscle of endurance athletes: Effect of L-carnitine. *Biochem Biophys Res Commun* 1992; 188: 102-106.

[46] McCarty MF. Promotion of hepatic lipid oxidation and gluconeogenesis as a strategy for appetite control. *Medical Hypotheses* 1994; 42: 215-225.

[47] Kaats G et al. The short-term therapeutic efficacy of treating obesity with a plan of improved nutrition and moderate caloric restriction. *Curr Ther Res* 1992; 51 (2): 261-274.

[48] Zhi-Qian He et al. Body weight reduction in adolescents by a combination of measures including using L-carnitine. *Acta Nutrimenta Sinica* 1997; 19(2): 146-151.

[49] Jeppesen J et al. Effects of low-fat, high-carbohydrate diets on risk factors for ischemic heart disease in postmenopausal women. *Am J Clin Nutr* 1997; 65: 1027-1033.

[50] Wolfe BM. Potential role of raising dietary protein intake for reducing risk of atherosclerosis. *Canadian Journal of Cardiology* 1995; 11 (Supplement G): 127G-131G.

[51] Ornish D et al. Can lifestyle changes reverse coronary heart disease? The lifestyle heart trial. *Lancet* 1990; 336: 129-133.

[52] Eaton SB, Eaton SB III, Konner MJ. Paleolithic nutrition revisited: A twelve-year retrospective on its nature and implications. *European Journal of Clinical Nutrition* 1997; 51: 207-216.

[53] Witte J et al. Diet and premenopausal bilateral breast cancer: A case control study. *Breast Cancer Research and Treatment* 1997; 42: 243-251.

[54] Godfrey K et al. Maternal nutrition in early and late pregnancy in relation to placental and fetal growth. *British Medical Journal* 1996; 312: 410-414.

[55] Holman P. Treating the ectomorphic constitution. *Journal of Nutritional and Environmental Medicine* 1996; 6: 359-370.

[56] Blackburn GL. Protein requirements with very low-calorie diets. *Postgrad Med J* 1984; 60 Suppl 3: 59-65.

[57] Raloff J. How the brain knows when to stop eating. *Science News* 1996; 150, 343.

[58] Hunt J et al. High- versus low-meat diets: Effects on zinc absorption, iron status, and calcium, copper, iron, magnesium, manganese, nitrogen, phosphorus, and zinc balance in postmenopausal women. *Amer J Clin Nutr* 1995; 62: 621-632.

[59] Spencer H, Kramer L. Factors contributing to osteoporosis. *Journal of Nutrition* 1986; 116: 316-319.

[60] Spencer H, Kramer L. Further studies of the effect of a high-protein diet as meat on calcium metabolism. *Amer J Clin Nutr* 1983; 37(6): 924-929.

[61] Cooper C et al. Dietary protein and bone mass in women. *Calcified Tissue International* 1996; 58: 320-325.

[62] McIntosh G et al. Dietary proteins protect against dimethylhydrazine-induced intestinal cancers in rats. *Journal of Nutrition* 1995; 125: 809-816.

[63] Scott FW. Food-induced type 1 diabetes in the BB rat. *Diabetes Metabolism Reviews* 1996; 12: 341-359.

[64] Coward L et al. Genistein, daidzein, and their beta-glycoside conjugates: Antitumor isoflavones in soybean food from Asian diets. *J Agric Food Chem* 1993; 41(11): 1961-1967.

[65] Lonnerdal B et al. The effect of individual components of soy formula and cows' milk formula on zinc bioavailability. *Amer J Clin Nutr* 1984; 40: 1064-1070.

[66] Sugiyama K et al. Methionine content of dietary proteins affects the molecular species composition of plasma phosphatidylcholine in rats fed a cholesterol-free diet. *Journal of Nutrition* 1997; 127: 600-607.

[67] Scrimshaw NS et al. Protein metabolism of young men during university examinations. *Am J Clin Nutr* 1966; 18: 321-324.

[68] Lemon P. Is increased dietary protein necessary or beneficial for individuals with a physically active lifestyle? *Nutrition Reviews* 1996 (II), S169-S175.

[69] Ogle KA et al. Children with allergic rhinitis and/or bronchial asthma treated with elimination diet. *Annals of Allergy* 1977; 39:8-11.

[70] Weisselberg B et al. A lamb based formula for infants allergic to casein hydrolysate formulas. *Clinical Pediatrics* 1996; 35 (10) 491-495.

[71] Sandstead HH. Is zinc deficiency a public health problem in America? *Nutrition* 1995; 11(1 Suppl): 87-92.

[72] Ip C. Review of the effects of trans fatty acids, oleic acid, n-3 polyunsaturated fatty acids, and conjugated linoleic acid on mammary carcinogenesis in animals. *Am J Clin Nutr* 1997; 66 (suppl): 1523S-1529S.

[73] Frank B. *Nucleic acid nutrition and therapy.* New York: Rainstone, 1977.

[74] Storlein LH, Baur LA, Kriketos AD et al. Dietary fats and insulin action. *Diabetologia* 1996; 39: 621-631.

[75] Okuyama H, Kobayashi T, Watanabe S. Dietary fatty acids—the n-6/n-3 balance and chronic elderly diseases. Excess linoleic acid and relative n-3 deficiency seen in Japan. *Prog Lipid Res* 1997; 35 (4): 409-457.

[76] Delarue J et al. Effects of fish oil on metabolic responses to oral fructose and glucose loads in healthy humans. *American Journal of Physiology* 1996; 270: E353-E362.

[77] Okuno M et al. Perilla oil prevents the excessive growth of visceral adipose tissue in rats by down-regulating adipocyte differentiation. *Journal of Nutrition* 1997; 127:1752-1757.

[78] Storlien LH. Not all dietary fats may lead to obesity. *Amer J Clin Nutr* 1990; 51: 1114.

[79] Leyton J et al. Differential oxidation of saturated and unsaturated fatty acids in vivo in the rat. *British Journal of Nutrition* 1987; 57: 383-393.

[80] Cunnane SC et al. N-3 Essential fatty acids decrease weight gain in genetically obese mice. *British Journal of Nutrition* 1986; 56: 87-95.

[81] Hainault I et al. Fish oil in a high lard diet prevents obesity, hyperlipidemia, and adipocyte insulin resistance in rats. *Annals of the New York Academy of Sciences* 1993; 683: 98-101.

[82] Pan DA, Storlein LH. Dietary lipid profile is a determinant of tissue phospholipid fatty acid composition and rate of weight gain in rats. *Journal of Nutrition* 1993; 123: 512-519.

[83] Rossner S et al. Fatty acid composition in serum lipids and adipose tissue in severe obesity before and after six weeks of weight loss. *International Journal of Obesity* 1989; 13 (5): 603-612.

[84] Storlien L et al. The type of dietary fat has a profound influence on development of insulin resistance in rats. *Diabetes Res Clin Pract* 1988; 5 (suppl 1): S267.

[85] Davis AT, Davis PG, Phinney SD. Plasma and urinary carnitine of obese subjects on very-low-calorie diets. *Journal of the American College of Nutrition* 1990; 9: 261-264.

[86] Birkhahn R et al. Potential of the monoglyceride and triglyceride of DL-3-hydroxybutyrate for parenteral nutrition: Synthesis and preliminary biological testing in the rat. *Nutrition* 1997; 13: 213-219.

[87] Prasad AN et al. Alternative epilepsy therapies: the ketogenic diet, immunoglobulins, and steroids. *Epilepsia* 1996; 37(suppl 1): S81-S95.

[88] Nebeling LC et al. Effects of a ketogenic diet on tumor metabolism and nutritional status in pediatric oncology patients: Two case reports. *Journal of the American College of Nutrition* 1995; 14 (2): 202-208.

[89] Nebeling LC, Lerner E. Implementing a ketogenic diet based on medium-chain triglyceride oil in pediatric patients with cancer. *Journal of the American Dietetic Association* 1995; 95 (6): 693-697.

[90] Phinney SD et al. The human metabolic response to chronic ketosis without caloric restriction: Preservation of submaximal exercise capability with reduced carbohydrate oxidation. *Metabolism* 1983; 32 (8): 769-776.

[91] Natali A et al. Effects of acute hypercarnitinemia during increased fatty acid substrate oxidation in Man. *Metabolism* 1993; 42(5): 594-600.

[92] Tillotson JL. Food group and nutrient intakes at baseline in the Multiple Risk Factor Intervention Trial. *Am J Clin Nutr* 1997; 65(1 Suppl): 228S-257S.

[93] De Oliveira e Silva ER et al. Effects of shrimp consumption on plasma lipoproteins. *Am J Clin Nutr* 1996; 64(5):712-717.

[94] Mann D. Purple grape juice, wine and beer all cardioprotective. *Medical Tribune*, May 1, 1997; 26.

[95] Lavin JH et al. The effect of sucrose- and aspartame-sweetened drinks on energy intake, hunger and food choice of female, moderately restrained eaters. *Int J Obes Relat Metab Disord* 1997; 21(1): 37-42.

[96] Enig M. Health and nutritional benefits from coconut oil and its advantages over competing oils. *Price-Pottenger Nutrition Foundation Journal* 1996; 20: 3-5.

[97] Prior IA et al. Cholesterol, coconuts, and diet on Polynesian atolls: A natural experiment: The Pukapuka and Tokelau island studies. *Am J Clin Nutr* 1981; 34: 1552-1561.

[98] Watanabe SW et al. Effects of L- and DL-carnitine on patients with impaired exercise tolerance. *Japanese Heart Journal* 1995; 36: 319-331.

[99] Geliebter A et al. Effects of strength or aerobic training on body composition, resting metabolic rate, and peak oxygen consumption in obese dieting subjects. *Am J Clin Nutr* 1997; 66: 557-563.

[100] Seppa N. High blood pressure can shrink the brain. *Science News* 1997; 152: 22.

[101] Patti, F. et al. Effects of L-acetylcarnitine on functional recovery of hemiplegic patients. *Clinical Trials Journal* 1988; 25 (Supp 1), 87-101.

[102] Amenta F et al. Reduced lipofuscin accumulation in senescent rat brain by long-term acetyl-L-carnitine treatment. *Arch Gerontol Geriatr* 1989; 9(2):147-153.

[103] Kohjimoto Y et al. Effects of acetyl-L-carnitine on the brain lipofuscin content and emotional behavior in aged rats. *Jpn J Pharmacol* 1988; 48(3): 365-371.

[104] Rampello L et al. Trophic action of acetyl-L-carnitine in neuronal cultures. *Acta Neurol* (Napoli) 1992;14(1):15-21.

[105] Gadaleta MN et al. Reduced transcription of mitochondrial DNA in the senescent rat. Tissue dependence and effect of L-carnitine. *Eur J Biochem* 1990; 187(3):501-506.

[106] Aureli T et al. Aging brain: Effect of acetyl-L-carnitine treatment on rat brain energy and phospholipid metabolism. A study by 31P and 1H NMR spectroscopy. *Brain Research* 1990; 526(1):108-112.

[107] McEwen BS et al. Neuroendocrine aspects of cerebral aging. *Int J Clin Pharm Res* 1990; 10: 7-14.

[108] Brierley EJ, Johnson MA, James OF, Turnbull DM. Effects of physical activity and age on mitochondrial function. *QJM* 1996; 89(4): 251-258.

[109] Fernandez C, Proto C. L-carnitine in the treatment of chronic myocardial ischemia. An analysis of 3 multicenter studies and a bibliographic review. *Clin Ter* 1992; 140 (4): 353-377.

[110] Regitz V et al. Defective myocardial carnitine metabolism in congestive heart failure secondary to dilated cardiomyopathy and to coronary, hypertensive and valvular heart diseases. *Am J Cardiol* 1990 ; 65(11): 755-760.

[111] Kobayashi A, Masumura Y, Yamazaki N. L-carnitine treatment for congestive heart failure—experimental and clinical study. *Japan Circulation Journal* 1992; 56 (1): 86-94.

[112] Johnston C. Comparison of the absorption and excretion of three commercially available sources of vitamin C. *Journal of the American Dietetic Association* 1994; 94(7): 779-781.

[113] Veronique A et al. High-density lipoprotein subfractions as markers of early atherosclerosis. *Am J Cardiol* 1995; 75: 127-131.

[114] Pola P et al. Carnitine in the therapy of dyslipidemic patients. *Curr Ther Res* 1980; 27: 208.

[115] Plioplys AV, Plioplys S. Serum levels of carnitine in chronic fatigue syndrome: Clinical correlates. *Neuropsychobiology* 1995; 32 (3): 132-138

[116] Plioplys AV, Plioplys S. Amantadine and L-carnitine treatment of chronic fatigue syndrome. *Neuropsychobiology* 1997; 35 (1): 16-23.

[117] Kuratsune H et al. Acylcarnitine deficiency in chronic fatigue syndrome. *Clinical Infectious Diseases* 1994; 18 (Supp 1): S 62-67.

[118] Plioplys AV, Bagherpour S, Kasnicka I. L-carnitine as a treatment of lethargy in children with chronic neurologic handicaps. *Brain Dev* 1994; 16 (2):146-149.

[119] Fulcher KY, White PD. Randomized controlled trial of graded exercise in patients with chronic fatigue syndrome. *British Medical Journal* 1997; 314: 1647-1652.

[120] Gecele M et al. Acetyl-L-carnitine in aged subjects with major depression: clinical efficacy and effects on the circadian rhythm of cortisol. *Dementia* 1991; 2: 333-337.

[121] Tempesta E et al. L-acetylcarnitine in depressed elderly subjects. A cross-over study versus placebo. *Drugs, Experimental and Clinical Research* 1987; 13(7): 417-423.

[122] Alpert J. Nutrition and depression: The role of folate. *Nutrition Reviews* 1997; 55 (5): 145-149.

[123] Cederblad G, Hermansson G, Ludvigsson J. Plasma and urine carnitine in children with diabetes mellitus. *Clin Chim Acta* 1982; 125(2):207-217.

[124] Paulson D, Shug A. The beneficial effects of L-carnitine in diabetes mellitus. *Proc Fed Am Soc Exper Biol* 1982; 41: 1087(abstract).

[125] Heller W et al. Effect of L-carnitine on post-stress metabolism in surgical patients. *Infusionsther Klin Ernahr* 1986; 13 (6): 268-276.

[126] Harper P et al. Increased liver carnitine content in obese women. *Am J Clin Nutr* 1995; 61: 18-25.

[127] Capaldo B et al. Carnitine improves peripheral glucose disposal in non-insulin-dependent diabetic patients. *Diabetes Res Clin Pract* 1991; 14 (3): 191-195.

[128] Paulson DJ, Sanjak M, Shug AL. Carnitine deficiency in the diabetic heart. In *Current Concepts in Carnitine Research*, ed. AL Carter. Boca Raton: CRC Press, 1992: 215-230.

[129] Rodrigues B, Xiang H, McNeill JH et al. Effect of L-carnitine treatment on lipid metabolism and cardiac performance in chronically diabetic rats. *Diabetes* 1988; 37: 1358-1364.

[130] Feuvray D, Idell-Wegner JA, Neely NR. Effects of ischemia on rat myocardial function and metabolism in diabetes. *Circ Res* 1979; 44: 322-329.

[131] Lowitt S et al. Acetyl-L-carnitine corrects the altered peripheral nerve function of experimental diabetes. *Metabolism* 1995; 44(5): 677-680.

[132] Gorio A et al. Peptide alterations in autonomic diabetic neuropathy prevented by acetyl-L-carnitine. *Int J Clin Pharmacol Res* 1992; 12: 225-230.

[133] O'Dea K. Marked improvement in carbohydrate and lipid metabolism in diabetic Australian aborigines after temporary reversion to traditional lifestyle. *Diabetes* 1984; 33: 596-604.

[134] Zhou B et al. The relationship of dietary animal protein and electrolytes to blood pressure: A study on 3 three Chinese populations. *International Journal of Epidemiology* 1994; 23 (4): 716-722.

[135] De Simone C et al. L-carnitine deficiency in AIDS patients. *AIDS* 1992; 6 (2): 203-205

[136] DeSimone C et al. High dose L-carnitine improves immunologic and metabolic parameters in AIDS patients. *Immunopharmacology and Immunotoxicology*, 1993; 15:1-2.

[137] Semino-Mora, MC et al. The effect of L-carnitine on the AZT-induced destruction of human myotubes. *Laboratory Investigation* 1994; 71 (5): 773-781.

[138] Dalakas, M et al. Zidovudine-induced mitochondrial myopathy is associated

with muscle carnitine deficiency and lipid storage. *Annals of Neurology* 1994; 35 (4): 482-487.

[139] Cossarizza A. Mitochondria alterations and dramatic tendency to undergo apoptosis in peripheral blood lymphocytes during acute HIV syndrome. *AIDS* 1997 Jan; 11(1):19-26

[140] Cifone MG et al. Effect of L-carnitine treatment in vivo on apoptosis and ceramide generation in peripheral blood lymphocytes from AIDS patients. *Proc Assoc Am Physicians* 1997;109 (2): 146-153

[141] De Simone C. Carnitine depletion in peripheral blood mononuclear cells from patients with AIDS: effect of oral L-carnitine. *AIDS* 1994; 8 (5): 655-660

[142] De Simone C, Calvani M. Acetyl-L-carnitine as a modulator of the neuro-endocrine-immune interaction in HIV+ subjects. In *Stress and Immunity and Aging: A Role for Acetyl-L-Carnitine*, New York: Elsevier, 1989, 125-138.

[143] Maebashi M et al. Lipid-lowering effect of carnitine in patients with type IV hyperlipoproteinemia. *Lancet* 1978; 2: 805.

[144] Slonim A et al. Non-ketotic hypoglycemia: An early indicator of systemic carnitine deficiency. *Neurology* 1983; 33: 29-33.

[145] Perros P et al. Brain abnormalities demonstrated by magnetic resonance imaging in Adult IDDM patients with and without a history of recurrent severe hypoglycemia. *Diabetes Care* 1997; 20(6): 1013-1017.

[146] Stenson J. Many thyroid problems are undiagnosed. *Medical Tribune* 1996: 2.

[147] Maebashi M et al. Urinary excretion of carnitine in patients with hyperthyroidism and hypothyroidism: Augmentation by thyroid hormone. *Metabolism* 1977; 21: 351-356.

[148] Maebashi M, Imamura A, Yoshinaga K. Effect of aging on lipid and carnitine metabolism. *Tohoku J Exp Med* 1982; 138(2):231-236.

[149] Rebouche C, Paulson D. Carnitine metabolism and function in humans. *Annual Review of Nutrition* 1986; 6: 41-66.

[150] Franceschi C, Cossarizza A, Troiano L, Salati R, Monti D. Immunological parameters in aging: Studies on natural immunomodulatory and immunoprotective substances. *Int J Clin Pharmacol Res* 1990; 10(1-2): 53-57.

[151] Keskin S et al. Could L-carnitine be an acute energy inducer in catabolic conditions? *Dev Med Child Neurol* 1997; 39 (3): 174-177.

[152] Borum P. Carnitine. *Annual Review of Nutrition* 1983; 3: 233-259.

[153] Brevetti G et al. Increases in walking distance in patients with peripheral vascular disease treated with L-carnitine: A double-blind, crossover study. *Circulation* 1988; 77: 767-773.

[154] Brevetti G et al. Carnitine-related alterations in patients with intermittent claudication. Indication for a focused carnitine therapy. *Circulation* 1996; 93: 1685-1689.

[155] Chanda S, Mehendale H et al. Role of nutritional fatty acid and L-carnitine in

the final outcome of thioacetamide hepatotoxicity. *FASEB Journal* 1994; 8: 1061-1068.

[156] Fiore L, Rampello L. L-acetylcarnitine attenuates the age-dependent decrease of NMDA-sensitive glutamate receptors in rat hippocampus. *Acta Neurol* (Napoli) 1989; 11(5):346-350.

[157] Passeri M et al. Mental impairment in aging: Selection of patients, methods of evaluation and therapeutic possibilities of acetyl-L-carnitine. *Int J Clin Pharmacol Res* 1988; 8(5):367-376.

[158] Patacchioli FR et al. Acetyl-L-carnitine reduces the age-dependent loss of glucocorticoid receptors in the rat hippocampus: An autoradiographic study. *J Neurosci Res* 1989; 23(4): 462-466.

[159] Ghirardi O et al. Effect of long-term acetyl-L-carnitine on stress-induced analgesia in the aging rat. *Exp Gerontol* 1994; 29(5):569-574.

[160] De Angelis C et al. Levocarnitine acetyl stimulates peripheral nerve regeneration and neuromuscular junction remodeling following sciatic nerve injury. *Int J Clin Pharmacol Res* 1992; 12: 269-279.

[161] Fernandez E, Pallini R, Tamburrini G et al. Effects of levo-acetylcarnitine on second motoneuron survival after axotomy. *Neurol Res* 1995; 17 (5): 373-376.

[162] De Grandis D et al. L-Acetylcarnitine in the treatment of patients with peripheral neuropathies. *Clin Drug Invest* 1995; 10 (6): 317-322.

[163] Rasmusson DX et al. Head injury as a risk factor in Alzheimer's disease. *Brain Injury* 1995; 9 (3): 213-219.

[164] Pettegrew J et al. Clinical and neurochemical effects of acetyl-L-carnitine in Alzheimer's disease. *Neurobiology of Aging* 1995; 16(1): 1-4.

[165] Spagnoli A et al. Long-term acetyl-L-carnitine treatment in Alzheimer's disease. *Neurology* 1991; 41: 1726-1732.

[166] Carta A et al. Acetyl-L-carnitine and Alzheimer's disease: Pharmacological considerations beyond the cholinergic sphere. *Ann N Y Acad Sci* 1993; 695:324-326.

[167] Hadjivassiliou M et al. Does cryptic gluten sensitivity play a part in neurological illness? *Lancet* 1996; 347: 369-371.

[168] Bodis-Wollner, I et al. Acetyl-levo-carnitine protects against MPTP-induced Parkinsonism in primates. *Journal of Neural Transmission* 1991; 3: 63-72.

[169] Sershen H et al. Effect of acetyl-L-carnitine on the dopaminergic system in aging brain. *J Neurosci Res* 1991; 30(3):555-559.

[170] Genazzani AD et al. Acetyl-L-carnitine as possible drug in the treatment of hypothalamic amenorrhea. *Acta Obstet Gynecol Scand* 1991; 70: 1-6.

[171] Virmani MA et al. Effects of L-acetylcarnitine on the pituitary-gonadal axis in female rats. International Symposium on Major Advances in Human Female Reproduction, Universita Catolica, Rome, 1990.

[172] Matsuda I, Ohtani Y. Carnitine status in Reye and Reye-like syndromes. *Pediatr Neurol* 1986; 2(2):90-94.

[173] Lolic MM, Fiskum G, Rosenthal RE. Neuroprotective effects of acetyl-L-carnitine after stroke in rats. *Ann Emerg Med* 1997; 29(6):758-765.

[174] Bohles H et al. The effect of preoperative L-carnitine supplementation on myocardial metabolism during aorto-coronary-bypass surgery. *Curr Ther Res* 1986; 39: 429-435.

[175] Fabbri G et al. Aging modifies the hormonal responses in women. *Neuroendocrine Letters* 1989; 11:4.

[176] Shuaib A, Waqaar T, Wishart T, Kanthan R, Howlett W. Acetyl-L-carnitine attenuates neuronal damage in gerbils with transient forebrain ischemia only when given before the insult. *Neurochem Res* 1995; 20(9):1021-1025.

[177] Griffin K. They should have washed their hands. *Hippocrates*, February 1997; 50-56.

[178] Triglycerides increase heart disease. *Nutrition Week* 1996; 26 (47): 7.

[179] Mensink RP, Katan MB. Effect of dietary fatty acids on serum lipids and lipoproteins. A meta-analysis of 27 trials. *Arterioscler Thromb* 1992; 12: 911-919.

[180] Fukagawa NK et al. High-carbohydrate, high-fiber diets increase peripheral insulin sensitivity in healthy young and old adults. *Am J Clin Nutr* 1990; 52 (3): 524-528.

[181] Etzioni A et al. Systemic carnitine deficiency exacerbated by a strict vegetarian diet. *Arch Dis Child* 1984; 59(2): 177-179.

INDEX

blood cholesterol. *See* cholesterol; HDL
cholesterol; LDL cholesterol
blood sugar imbalances, 47
bone loss, 92
brain, 150-153
   carnitine and function of, 27
   effects of stress on, 162-165
   fats for, 151
   herbs for, 151
   maximizing health of, 152-153
   mental exercises and health of, 153
   nutrients for, 150-151
   questions about acetyl-L-carnitine,
     157-158
   slowing aging with acetyl-L-carnitine,
     154-156
   supplements for, 152, 199, 201-203
bread and cereal products
   on Carnitine Program, 139
   effects of, 47
   food allergies and, 86
   phytates in whole wheat bread, 34
breakfast
   cottage cheese for, 143
   guidelines for, 113-114
breast cancer
   bread and cereal products and, 47
   high intake of carbohydrates and
     sweetened beverages, 85
Brindall berry (garcina extract), 147
bronchitis, 176

calcium
   Paleolithic and current intakes of, 33
   phytates' effect on absorption, 86
   protein intake and levels of, 92
   whole wheat consumption and, 34
calories, 110, 116
cancer
   benefits of carnitine for, 27
   breast, 47, 85
   colorectal, 47
   supplements for, 177-178
candida albicans
   food allergies and, 60
   high-carbohydrate diet and, 85
   treatment of, 178-180
   vegetarian diet and, 47
carbohydrates
   adding back after Phases I and II, 136,
     146
   amounts to eat, 138
   balancing intake of, 80

   at breakfast, 113
   on Carnitine Program, 116
   combining with fat, 43
   defined, 34
   dietary disadvantages of grains, 34
   food pyramid recommendations for, 39
   metabolizing with carnitine, 70, 72
   processed foods and lack of variation
     in, 35
   reasons to reduce, 85-86
   regaining weight and adding, 146
   sources of paleocarbs and neocarbs, 34
   suggested servings of, 84
   in vegetarian diet, 47
   yeast overgrowths and, 47
carnitine
   advantages of, 17-20
   benefits of, 26-27
   carnitine tartrate form of, 23-24, 68
   defined, 16
   energizing effects of, 66
   foods containing, 17
   with garcinia extract and chromiun
     picolate, 147
   infant nutrition and, 195-196
   ketosis-inducing diet and, 129
   in meat, 97
   metabolizing lactate, 70
   with other medications, 145
   questions about, 143-145
   reasons to take, 214-215
   recommended doses, 61, 76, 146-147
   for Reye's syndrome, 208
   slowing aging with, 28-30
   source of supplements, 144
   sports performance and, 68-72
   taking acetyl-L-carnitine or, 144
   for weight loss, 23, 73-78
   when benefits appear, 144
   when to take, 71, 76
   see also acetyl-L-carnitine; carnitine
     tartrate; L-carnitine; nutrients and
     supplements
Carnitine Program, 108-110
   adding more carnitine, 146-147
   breaks on, 117
   common questions about, 138-145
   eating out and, 118-119
   exercise and, 147
   fats on, 147
   food allergies, 148
   garcinia extract and chromiun pico-
     late, 147

digesting protein, 90
dinner guidelines, 114
disease
    preventing with carnitine, 17-18
    see also specific diseases listed individ-
        ually
DL-Carnitine, 144

eating out, 118-119
emotions
    energy and, 60
    relating to food, 24-25
endurance
    carnitine tartrate for athletic, 68
    increasing, 68-69, 72
energy
    antiaging force of, 28
    benefits of carnitine on, 26
    with carnitine intake, 17-18
    maximizing, 59-60
    natural vs. stimulant, 65-67
    nutrients for cells and, 56-58
    nutrients maximizing, 61-64
    oxygen as source of, 29
    protein intake and, 89
energy therapy, 168-171
    dietary suggestions for, 170-171
    exercises and, 170
    principles of, 168-170
environment and meat industry, 96
EPA fats, 57, 151, 159
ephedra (Ma Huang), 66-67, 153
epilepsy, 158
Epsom salt baths, 152
Ester C, 177-178
exercise
    adjusting food intake to, 116
    with Carnitine Program, 147
    carnitine's effects on, 68, 69, 70-71
    energy therapy and, 170
    maximizing brain health and, 152
    maximizing energy with, 59
    metabolizing lactate, 70
    permanent weight loss and, 76-77
    protein intake and, 90
    proteins needs and, 94

fat, body
    balancing in blood and cells, 18-19
    carnitine's role in burning, 21, 68, 72
    combining with carbohydrates, 43
    food pyramid recommendations for,
        38

in Paleolithic diet, 42
in weight-loss diet, 80
fat-free diets, 75-76
fatigue
    chronic, 27, 182-184
    medical conditions leading to, 60
fats, dietary
    for brain nutrition, 151
    on Carnitine Program, 147
    for Phase I, 111
    questions about cooking with, 142
    types of, 100
    using omega-3, 75
    see also oils; omega-3 fats
Felix Letter, The, 219
fiber, 33, 34-35
fibromyalgia
    benefits of carnitine on, 27
    treating, 183-184
flaxmeal
    making, 120
    sources of, 132
    using in shakes, 114
flaxseed oil
    as cell energizer, 57
    combining with vegetable oils, 100-101
    recommended doses for, 62
    response to insulin and, 100
    in salad dressings, 120
flaxseeds, 132
folic acid, 62, 159
food allergies
    candida albicans and, 60
    dairy products and, 97
    grains and, 86
    maximizing energy and, 59
    seasonal variety in foods and, 43
    weight gain and, 148
food cravings
    in high carbohydrate diet, 47
    protein intake and, 90
food pyramid
    animal products from grass-fed ani-
        mals, 39-40
    biochemical individuality and, 40
    carbohydrates on, 39
    dairy products in, 40
    development of, 37-40
    fats, starches, and antinutrients in, 38-
        39
    individualized needs in diet, 39
    nutritional variation and, 39
    protein in, 39-40

CoQ10, 61
  for depression, 185-186
  energy and, 56-58, 61-64
  for energy therapy, 171
  flaxseed oil, 62
  for healthy balance of cholesterol,
     181-182
  for heart health, 173
  for high blood pressure, 189
  for hyperthyroidism, 192-194
  for hypoglycemia, 192
  for immune system enhancement,
     194-195
  increasing for energy, 60
  for intermittent claudication, 197-198
  lipoic acid, 63
  for liver, 198-199
  for lowering triglycerides, 211-212
  magnesium, 62
  malic acid, 62-63
  in meat, 95-98
  medium chain triglycerides (MCTs),
     57, 63
  for memory enhancement, 199
  for mitral valve prolapse, 200
  for muscle tension, 200-201
  NADH, 64
  omega-3 fats and key supplements, 103
  optimal needs for, 50-51
  for Parkinson's disease, 206-207
  preparing body for surgery, 209-210
  stimulants vs. natural energizing, 65-67
  for stroke, 208-209
  therapeutic foods for weight loss, 213
  for treatment of infertility, 196-197
  for vegetarian diet, 21, 212
  vitamin C, 63
  vitamin E, 63
  weight loss and, 74, 213
nutritional variation
  missing on food pyramid, 39
  need for, 35
  on Paleolithic diet, 44
nuts and seeds, 88, 137

obesity
  preventing with omega-3 oils, 100-101
  protein and, 93
  psychological causes for, 24-25
oils
  coconut, 142
  fighting obesity and, 100-101
  flaxseed, 57, 62, 100-101, 120

MCT, 132
  saturated fats with omega-3, 100-101
  suggested for Carnitine Program, 137
  see also omega-3 fats
olives, 137
omega-3 fats, 99-104
  adding on Carnitine Program, 116
  combining saturated fats with, 100-101
  dietary advantages of, 100
  dieting and loss of, 101-103
  grass-fed animal products and, 39-40
  from meats, 97
  preventing insulin resistance, 100, 104
  promoting use of, 105-107
  sources of, 23, 75
  in vegetarian diet, 47
omega-6 fats, 47, 106
optimal health, 53-55
  defined, 50-52
  energizing nutrients for, 61-64
  need for, 49-50
organic foods for Paleolithic diet, 43
Ornish, Dr. Dean, 81

Paleodiet Symposium Archive, The, 220
Paleolithic diet, 41-44
  ancestral needs and, 44
  animal products on, 42-43
  for children, 96
  combining fat and carbohydrates, 43
  fat and, 42
  foods and food preparation for, 42-43
  grain and dairy products for, 42-43
  high blood pressure and, 189
  low carbohydrate diet and, 82
  nutritional variation on, 44
  similarities between ketogenic diet
     and, 130
Paleolithic food pyramid, 31, 32, 33
Parkinson's disease
  NADH and, 64
  pesticides and, 153
  supplements for, 206-207
pasta, 140-141
patience and weight loss, 77
pesticides, 153
Phase I. See Carnitine Program Phase I
Phase II. See Carnitine Program Phase II
phosphatidyl choline, 160, 163
phosphatidyl serine, 152, 159
phytates
  effect on absorption of calcium and
     zinc, 86